MORE
or
Less?

Dedicated to Michelle Obama, America's First Lady of Physical Fitness, who is leading the fight against childhood obesity, by her personal example and dedicated promotion of her 'Let's move' health campaign.

MORE

or

Less?

Discover the Secrets of

Lifetime

Weight Control

Donald Norfolk

Self Help Alliance Ltd

This book offers a new approach to lifetime weight control, a programme which is easy to understand, fun to follow and permanent in its effects. Follow the 39-Step Programme and you'll gain a whole raft of spin-off benefits, as well as losing your superfluous weight. For instance, you'll have:

More physical attractiveness. Losing weight is the cheapest way of ensuring that you always look your best. Psychologists have found that when we meet strangers it takes them only ninety seconds to form their first impression, a judgement which is largely based on the way we look.

Less eye-catching unsightly blemishes which mar your natural healthy looks – like chubby cheeks, flabby thighs and a bulging belly.

More bounce to the ounce. The less surplus weight you carry the livelier you'll become.

Less fatigue and general ennui. You can't be as fit as a fiddle if you're shaped like a double bass. When people are four stone overweight they carry with them the equivalent of a half hundredweight sack of potatoes wherever they go. This explains why they get out of breath when they climb a short flight of stairs. Surveys show that people who are ten per cent overweight are twice as likely to suffer symptoms of breathlessness and chronic tiredness.

More chance of adding life to your years and years to your life. Surveys show that people who shed their excess weight increase their life expectancy by an average of four years.

Less risk of suffering premature death and crippling illnesses like hypertension, strokes, myocardial infarction, cancer and type 2 diabetes. If you carry excess weight you become your own executioner, a fate which is in keeping with the old adage: 'God sends the acute diseases, the chronic diseases we create ourselves'.

More mental agility and acumen. Brain scans show that people who maintain a healthy weight have a better blood flow to their brains than their overweight counterparts. This may improve their brain function, according to a team of researchers in Chicago who found that the less excess weight an over-sixty-year-old woman carries the better her memory and general brain function.

Less risk of dementia, according to research carried out in Sweden which revealed that people who put on weight in middle age are eighty per cent more likely to suffer dementia in later life.

Contents

Overture – and Beginners Please

The developed world is facing a life-threatening plague: a disaster of epidemic proportions which will kill far more people than the two world wars. After a sixty-year battle, we're finally winning the war against smoking. Now we must turn our attention to tackling the obesity epidemic, which is destined to take over from smoking as the world's major cause of preventable death. America, the world's wealthiest nation, spends twice as much per person on health care as Britain and most other European countries, and yet its health outcomes are decidedly poorer. The US suffers, not because of the poverty of its medical services, but because the great mass of its people follow an unhealthy lifestyle. That's the basic cause of the worldwide obesity plague. Unless positive action is taken, the future looks bleak. No country in the developed world will be able to finance its mounting health care costs, unless practical steps are taken to overcome the obesity plague.

The Way Forward

Thanks to the tireless endeavours of scientists from across the globe, we now know enough to stop the epidemic in its tracks. What we must do from this moment onwards is to make practical use of the knowledge they have amassed. It was easy for doctors to help their patients overcome their addiction to cigarettes. All they had to say was 'stop smoking', and maybe toss in one or two crutches like nicotine patches and herbal cigarettes. But you can't tell overweight people to 'stop eating'. To get meaningful long-term results doctors, and other health professionals, need to take on the role of personal trainers, and conduct each of their fat patients on a journey of personal lifestyle change. This they generally can't do, because of the time constraints under which they work. This book has been written to fill this gap, to collate the wealth of information which is now available about the causes of obesity and its cure, and to weld this into a simple programme of step-by-step lifestyle changes. If you're overweight, there's no call for you to become a fitness fanatic, food freak or health bore. There's no need to pump iron, run marathons, balance on your head or take endless five-day cleansing fasts. All that's required is that you should make a series of small changes in your daily routine, a process which St Theresa called the 'little way', and which educationalists today refer to as 'incremental learning'.

If we, as individuals, don't take immediate steps to tackle this crisis there's a very real risk that politicians will intervene. And that's where the troubles will really start, for there's no problem known to man which can't be made worse by government intervention. Even in the days of ancient Greece, the Spartan authorities introduced a decree which forced young men to line up in the nude for a physical inspection. Those who showed signs of putting on weight were forced to undergo a programme of strenuous physical exercise. A similar measure was recommended in East Germany, before the country's reunification, when the communist government proposed to reduce the social benefits of anyone who was overweight, on the grounds that they were costing the nation far too much in needless medical treatment and reduced industrial output. Since then, penalties have been imposed on overweight personnel in the police and armed services, and some private institutions are now imposing similar penalties and 'fat fines'. In 1978 the Oral Roberts University, a charismatic Christian institution in Texas, celebrated for its athletic prowess, began to suspend students for being too fat and failing to lose weight in a given period of time. Similar action has been taken by the Alabama Employees Insurance Board, which has approved a plan to charge obese workers $25 dollars a month if they don't take steps to reduce their weight and improve their health. This premium loading is fully justified, for a study of employees working at Duke University revealed that staff members who were morbidly obese made twice as many compensation claims, and had twelve times the levels of sickness absenteeism, as those who maintained a healthy weight.

The UK government has recently begun to issue statements suggesting that people must change their lifestyle if they want to lose weight. On that we can all agree, but at a time when our personal freedoms are being eroded, the last thing we want is for a nanny state to tell us how we should lead our lives. If we're overweight, we must accept that the fault is wholly ours, and likewise the responsibility for its cure. Instead we often close our eyes, and refuse to admit that we have a problem. Men who can't get into a bath at the same time as the water will refuse to admit that they're overweight. So too their wives, who, when waddling down the road may look like two little boys fighting under a blanket, yet still refuse to admit that they might be a tad too heavy. People blame their genes, but there's no evidence whatsoever that there's been any change in our genetic make-up over the last thirty years, which have witnessed a vast increase in the obesity figures. Even if your parents were lifelong members of the chubby, tubby club, it doesn't mean that *you* have to be fat.

Time for Change

I don't know how you came by this book – whether it was begged, borrowed, bought or stolen – but since it's in your hands at this moment I can only assume that you either realize that you have a weight problem, which you want to overcome, or you're a health professional, anxious to play your part in offering help to those in need. Whatever category you're in, we share the same goal, which is to find a reliable, scientifically based way of solving the obesity problem. The objective of this book is to provide that solution. Although it ploughs a totally new furrow, it's backed by a wealth of scientific evidence.

In some ways *More or Less?* is my response to the obscene news that there are now more people in the world crippled by obesity than suffering the effect of starvation and diseases linked with malnutrition. It represents the accumulation of over fifty years' work, an interest which started in the early 1950s, when a growing number of my patients asked my advice on how they could lose weight. As this demand became more insistent, I began to study the science of girth control in greater depth, and started to offer more general advice through my books, radio broadcasts and newspaper articles. This culminated in the publication of *The Habits of Health*, a self help guide which laid down the principles which form the basis of this book. In its introduction, I quoted Henry James, one of the founding fathers of modern psychotherapy, who said that by the age of twenty-five we are all a 'bundle of habits'. With their aid, we can spend a large part of our lives working on automatic pilot, doing things like brushing our hair without giving them a moment's conscious thought.

These habits have been learned, which means that they can equally well be unlearnt. But that reversal takes time, as was shown when a group of nearly a hundred American undergraduates was asked to select an activity which they thought might improve their health. One thought he'd benefit by taking a fifteen-minute run before dinner, another to eat a piece of fruit with lunch, and a third to do fifty sit-ups during his morning coffee break. The subjects were then asked to repeat these health-related behaviours for the next twelve weeks, the object of the trial being to see how long it would take them to make these activities a habitual part of their daily routine. This proved to be subject to widespread variation, but on average the practices became part of their automatic default setting after a period of about ten weeks. Clearly beneficial change is possible, for anyone who has the patience and persistence to bring it about.

This book offers you a timed programme, incorporating thirty-nine steps, each of which will help you groove an enhanced lifestyle. With their aid you'll lose weight, restore the supremacy of your body's inherent weight controlling mechanism, and gain a cornucopia of additional health benefits.

There's a well-known Chinese saying: 'Give a man a fish and you feed him for a day. Teach him how to fish and you feed him for a lifetime.' In the context of this book, that adage could be paraphrased to read: 'Give an overweight person a diet sheet and you'll help them lose weight for a few weeks. Help them to change their habits, and you'll keep them fit for an entire lifetime.' Every day we're faced with an endless array of choices. Most of these are trivial, like deciding on which side to put the butter on a slice of toast, but others are absolutely vital to our well-being. It's these we need to monitor. We often excuse ourselves by saying we're *creatures* of habit, forgetting that we're also *creators* of habits. Once we've worked to groove an array of sensible habits, we can then sit back and let our habits work for us.

The word 'diet' is derived from the Latin *diaita*, which originally meant a person's habitual manner of living, and not just a daily record of their food intake. If you want to achieve effortless, lifetime weight control you won't get far if you merely fiddle with your diet. What you need is a radical change in your way of life. So from now onwards, don't diet – *diaita*. That's an affirmation you'd do well to repeat from time to time in the coming months, until the habit changes you need to make have been firmly grooved. Psychologists involved in the process of behavioural change know how hard it is for people to alter their long-established habit patterns. This is largely because they must first extinguish the old, before they can establish the new. Just as ocean-going liners must empty their tanks before they take on a fresh supply of water, so we must extinguish our outmoded habits before we're capable of taking onboard a set of new, and more appropriate, behaviours. Whatever our age, we are all a work in progress. Any task becomes easy if it's tackled in a steady, progressive fashion, as is affirmed by the old Buddhist proverb: 'If you are facing in the right direction, all you need do is keep walking.' That's the process followed in this book. It's not an ascetic routine; it's about taking up rather than giving up, so if at any time it makes you feel miserable – you've got it wrong. Since the programme needs to be given a definitive name, I've chosen to call it the Slim Vitality programme, a term I've often used before. This will be shortened to EssVee, to make it slightly more distinctive. It offers a way of saying a final goodbye to your surplus fat, which is surely infinitely better than resorting to drugs, drastic dieting, liposuction or gastric surgery.

The Thirty-nine Steps
The idea for this book had a long gestation period, but its final form came in a sudden intuitive flash. I'd been poring over my notes and research files, trying to make some sense of the plethora of medical, psychological and biological data relating to weight control, and finally had an 'aha', or Eureka, moment. The epiphany came when I decided to compile a list of all the habits that needed to be changed in order to establish a healthy lifestyle. These would need to be mutually consistent, and capable of being linked together in an integrated programme. After a great deal of sorting, mixing and matching I finally ended up with thirty-nine separate steps, which just happens to be the allotted number of weeks for the development of a human foetus from conception to birth.

So now's the time to make up your mind. Don't waste time reading any more of this book if there's the slightest chance that you won't follow it through to its ultimate conclusion. To give up halfway would be like paying a hefty price to attend a concert performance of Beethoven's glorious Ninth Symphony and then quitting after the first movement and so missing the reward of the final, triumphant choral 'Ode to Joy'. It's never easy to bring about habit change, however strongly it's desired, but sometimes it's made easier by making a written declaration of intent. Experience shows that people who want to break their addiction to alcohol can be helped by signing a total abstinence pledge. In the same way, young girls who go to university, and want to remain chaste in a milieu filled with lusty adolescent males, often find their resolve is strengthened by making a solemn virginity pact. In the light of this experience, you might find it helpful to swear, sign and date the following simple oath: 'I pledge to devote the next nine months to following the EssVee programme of habit change and lifestyle weight control.' Once you've done that, tell your family, friends and colleagues of your resolve. Mark the date in your diary, or better still on a large and highly visible wall calendar, and then put a red ring around the same day in the thirty-nine weeks which follow. On each of those appointed days aim to read each week's assignment, a task which should take you no more than five minutes. Then write – or preferably type – in a large bold script a dozen or more copies of the brief summary which you'll find in the box at the end of each week's assignment. These should be distributed in places where they're most likely to be seen – on your office desk, above your computer, on the fridge door, attached to your bathroom mirror, taped to your bed, or fixed on the dashboard of your car.

Having done that, you're ready to move on to the course itself, bearing in mind that you'll get the best results if you spend an entire week mastering each step before you move on to the next. Health is a journey, not a destination, and in this case it will be a fun trip, for it will be a process not of denial but of life enhancement. This is for people who love to eat. So turn on. Get wise. Throw off your hair shirt and don your glad rags. And remember: **Don't diet** – *diaita*. Bon voyage!

STEP 1

The Shape of Things to Come

Welcome to the EssVee programme, which provides a totally new approach to lifetime weight control. The system is based on the very latest scientific evidence, drawn from research centres around the world. It's a user friendly approach, based on a process of gradual, incremental lifestyle change.

Every developed country today faces a massive obesity problem, a crisis which has arisen largely because we're following a dysfunctional way of life. During the last few decades every aspect of our lives has become increasingly ersatz. We've become denizens of an alien world, a realm full of artifice, contrivance and mechanization. As a result we've lost contact with the natural world and are now out of sync with the internal workings of our bodies. If we were not 'cribbed, cabined and confined' by the world around us, our bodies would take automatic care of our health. This they do through a series of intricate cybernetic arrangements programmed to maintain the optimum functioning of every one of our internal organs and vital activities. This process, collectively known as homeostasis, adjusts our blood pressure, body temperature and oxygen uptake according to our moment-to-moment needs. There's another complex homeostatic system, which we'll shortly describe in greater detail, which aims to regulate our food intake according to our exact nutritional needs. If we adopted a healthier lifestyle, this 'appestat' would ensure that we maintained a perfect balance between our energy needs and our energy intake. This is the mechanism which kept our ancestors slim and trim. The whole objective of the EssVee programme is to promote a healthy way of life which restores the primacy of the appestat mechanism.

Many of my patients claimed that they put on weight when they gave up smoking. Others said their figures ballooned when they were advised to take prescription drugs, or when they moved into the city and found it nigh on impossible to follow a healthy lifestyle. There's merit in all these excuses. Statistics show that people who quit smoking gain an average of ten to eleven pounds, slightly more for women than for men. In the same way, it's undoubtedly true that undesirable weight gain can be one of the side effects of certain medically prescribed drugs, such as steroids, anti-depressants and certain anticonvulsants. Surveys also show that if both your parents are fat, you're eight times as likely to be obese as when they're slim. Similarly in China, obesity is four times as high in cities as it is in the countryside. So, with some justification, you could easily spend your days justifying your excess avoirdupois. But that wouldn't solve your problem or boost your health. Nor would it prolong your life, for obese people reduce their life expectancy by an average of six to seven years. Even if you're a Chinese ex-smoker with two obese parents, living in Beijing and taking steroids to treat your asthma, you can still take steps to shed your excess pounds. Whatever your personal circumstances, you can choose whether you're fit or fat. From now onwards what you do, and what you are, is what you'll get.

This book could be a turning point in your life providing you admit that you have a problem and need help. It's a predicament which must be faced head on. It can't be swept under the carpet or hidden by wearing a larger pair of pants or a bell tent dress. Today you've reached a watershed. If you're overweight at present, and want to lead a long, productive life, you must at some point embark on an effective recovery programme, just as you would if you were an alcoholic or a heroin addict. Now is the time for you to begin that rehabilitation process. This is a task that only you can accomplish. This programme will work, only if you take the full responsibility for *making* it work. Just over fifty years ago Julian Rotter, a leading psychologist at Ohio State University, advanced the important concept of 'locus of control'. This is a technical term to describe the beliefs that people hold about the factors which influence their lives. According to Rotter's theory, some individuals believe that their destiny is determined by factors outside themselves. They're not to be blamed for their misfortunes. It's never their fault. It's fate, bad luck or the mistakes and thoughtless behaviour of other people. Rotter described these individuals as having an 'external locus of control', a world view often linked with feelings of insecurity, anxiety and depression. At the other end of the spectrum are those people who believe that the course of their life is largely determined by their own actions. They are defined as having an 'internal locus of control'. These individuals believe that they are masters of their own destiny, an outlook which imbues them with a sense of confidence and control. The step you must take this week is to take full responsibility for your long-term physical condition. Only losers believe in horoscopes, luck, lotteries and get-rich-quick schemes. You're a self-made person or you're nothing. That was the view of Bernard of Clairvaux, the twelfth-century monk, who said: 'No thing can work me damage but myself – I am never a real sufferer but by my own fault.'

You can permanently overcome your weight problem if you truly believe you can. This was shown when 7,500 Britons were followed from infancy until they reached their late thirties. The results revealed that children with a high internal locus of control not only had higher levels of self-esteem, but were also ten times less likely to be overweight at thirty than those who felt dependent on outside aid from doctors, dietitians, slimming aids and weight reducing pills. So don't pass the buck. Accept here and now that you, and you alone, are responsible for any overweight you carry. You don't *have* to adopt your parents' bad habits. Your father may have been a couch potato, but that doesn't mean that you must be equally idle. Similarly, there's no reason why you should follow your mother's example if she throughout her life was over fond of calorie-saturated doughnuts and hamburgers. If both your parents are overweight, take the responsibility for seeing that you're among the twenty-five per cent who don't follow their example. Many of my patients told me that they suffered from a hypoactive thyroid gland, which meant they were predestined to put on weight. In truth that's not the inevitable outcome, for more than half the people diagnosed with hypothyroidism are not over-weight. The only glands giving rise to the obesity epidemic that we face today are the salivary glands.

As far as our health is concerned, we are all self-made men and women. That was the key point made at the very start of Samuel Smile's highly influential book *Self Help*, which opened with the famous line: 'Heaven helps those who help themselves.' You can become the person you long to be, providing you modify your habits in a way which restores the primacy of your body's innate weight controlling mechanism.

STEP 1
Throughout this week I will confirm my commitment to the
EssVee programme, by reciting the words of the
English poet W. E. Henley:
'I am the master of my fate, I am the captain of my soul.'

STEP 2

Change Your Habits, Not Your Diet

You're reading this book because you want to lose weight. Maybe you were mortified to discover that you were having to struggle harder to put on your tights or socks, finding it was no longer easy to make both ends meet. Or, maybe, there was a dreadful moment when you tried to push yourself away from the table and only the table moved. Whatever the provocation, you're now about to shed those surplus pounds. This is a task you should approach with relish, coupled with a healthy dose of realism. It took several years to gain your surplus pounds, so it's unreasonable to expect that this excess weight can be shed in a few days. You court disappointment if you go on a crash diet in the hope that you'll be in shape for next month's beach holiday. It's not difficult to shed weight if you go on an unbalanced, low-calorie diet. Select whichever one takes your fancy, or is the most heavily hyped. One day the vogue will be for the Pritikin diet, the next for the Hollywood diet, the Grapefruit-only diet, the Atkins Diet or the fillet-steak-twice-a-day-straightway-to-bankruptcy diet. They have just one thing in common – they don't work. To begin with they trigger an impressive weight loss, but the lost pounds quickly return when a normal pattern of eating is resumed. Quite often, in fact, you'll find you're heavier than you were before the ordeal started. This was shown when researchers from the University of California reviewed thirty-one diet programmes and found that four or five years after a following a crash diet somewhere between a third and two-thirds of dieters weighed more than they did before they embarked on the diet. 'We concluded most of them would have been better off not going on the diet at all,' was the final judgement of Professor Traci Mann, the psychologist who led the study. Some try again and again with different diets, but with exactly the same results. Eventually they become victims of the yo-yo syndrome, suffering a succession of humiliating defeats as they struggle to keep slim on diets that are invariably unbalanced, boring, bland and anti-social.

This was true in the case of Oprah Winfrey, one of the many celebrities who've been a victim of yo-yo dieting, which one medical expert described as 'the rhythm method of weight control'. She shed five stone when she went on a low-calorie liquid protein diet. When it ended, she overate and quickly regained every ounce of the five stone she'd lost. She said her binge eating was the result of mental strain, when one of her peak time TV series was cancelled. But a nutritionist who knew her well pointed to the real problem. 'Oprah grew impatient. She tried to lose weight faster than her body could tolerate. If you stop eating you lose weight,' he explained, 'but when you return to eating, the problem – and causes that make you over-eat – are still there and you slip back into the same old ways.' The US impresario Billy Rose followed the 'if it tastes good spit it out regime'. He cut out all the foods he liked, and quickly lost twenty-five pounds, every ounce of which he regained the moment he returned to his normal pattern of eating.

Several studies have shown that it's more difficult to lose weight than to give up smoking if you rely on the old-fashioned ways of calorie counting and stringent food restriction. Millions have got themselves embroiled in this futile task, but only two per cent have maintained their weight loss for more than a few months. Crash dieting doesn't work, and the only people who benefit from wham-bam dieting are the 'experts' who write the diet books and the firms that sell the slimming foods. Those who follow stringent slimming diets are not only wasting their time, they're also taking unnecessary risks. Some, as a consequence, will suffer a deficiency of essential nutrients. A lack of body-building amino acids can arise if slimmers stop eating bread, which typically supplies a quarter of our total protein intake; and a similar shortage of calcium can occur if they reduce their intake of dairy foods. Furthermore, the sudden breakdown of adipose tissue floods the bloodstream with saturated fats, which can increase the risk of cardiovascular disease. This was confirmed by a 1991 study, published in the *New England Journal of Medicine*, which showed that people whose body weight drops too rapidly as a result of dieting show an increased risk of illness and death from coronary heart disease. Mario Lanza spent his life on an endless roller coaster ride of binge eating and crash dieting, once losing a hundred pounds in a brief spell of semi-starvation. As a result he suffered a heart attack and died at the age of thirty-eight. Rapid weight loss can also lead to the sudden release of toxins which are normally safely locked away in the body's fat stores. A ten-year study of over a thousand adults, carried out at the Kyungpook National University, South Korea, revealed that people who lost ten or more kilograms during the decade showed high levels of seventeen 'persistent organic pollutants'. These toxins enter the food chain from the absorption of environmental pesticides and toxic chemicals, and are known to predispose to cancer, dementia and diabetes.

The main thing you lose when you go on a low-calorie diet is your temper. Blood tests show that anyone who follows a standard one thousand calorie diet is likely to suffer a lowering of their blood levels of typtophan. This is a precursor of serotonin, the naturally occurring substance which raises the mood. As a result they're likely to feel a trifle depressed, which will often provoke them to comfort eat. Worst of all they may look a trifle haggard. This was the warning issued by the Harley Medical Group, who reported that a third of its female patients were seeking cosmetic surgery to cope with the skin changes caused by yo-yo dieting. As a company spokesperson explained: 'Continual weight change stretches the elastin in the skin which causes stretch marks to appear and deepens the look of those already on the skin.'

Rather than fight nature, we should work with her. Life is for living, not for counting calories or keeping a regular check on your weight and Body Mass Index. One of my friends was overweight and followed the complicated formula which enabled him to measure his BMI, and then went on a strict calorie counting diet, which he said was as about as exciting as kissing his grandmother. I saw him a few months later, and thought he looked harassed but not much trimmer. 'I haven't lost much weight,' he replied in answer to my query, 'but my mental arithmetic is far better than it was.' Eating gourmet food is one of life's great pleasures. So follow the EssVee programme. Don't diet – *diaita*.

> **STEP 2**
> This week I will show a greater appetite for life itself, and let quality rather than quantity determine the food I eat.

STEP 3

Mirror, Mirror on the Wall, Who's the Fairest of Them All?

Your motivation to follow the EssVee programme must be a matter of the heart as well as of the head. Will-power alone won't see you through. Most attempts to regain a healthy weight begin in the spring, when people look ahead to their summer holidays and the embarrassment of having to expose their overweight torsos to public gaze. Disgust is one of the major motivations which drives people to get slim. Terri Flaherty experienced a wave of self-loathing one April, when she left off her winter woollies and looked ahead to the seaside holiday she'd already booked. As a schoolgirl she'd worn a size ten swimsuit, now she was two stone heavier and could barely squeeze into one two sizes larger. 'I looked in the mirror and saw a chunky woman,' she recalls. The full-frontal sight of her naked body made her realize that something had to be done. The next day she started on a programme of lifestyle change – less processed foods, more exercise, and a switch to a diet rich in fruit and vegetables – and by the end of the year she'd shed the excess weight, and could comfortably get into size ten swimsuits. Quite by chance she discovered one of the finest of all slimming aids – a full-length bathroom mirror.

When researchers at the University of Texas questioned more than two thousand women about their body size, they discovered that fully a quarter of obese women considered themselves to be slim. Today that deception is easier to practise than ever before, for obesity is now the norm rather than the exception. But you still can't cheat a full-length mirror. This was shown some years ago when Albert Stunkard and Myer Mendelson, two doctors from the Penn-

16

sylvania Department of Psychiatry, got a large group of overweight patients to comment on what they saw when they viewed themselves in a full-length mirror. It was then they were forced to recognize their true plight. One woman told them: 'What I see is a big fat pig.' Another, who desperately wanted to get married, but realized her chances were slim because of her ungainly size, said: 'Who'd want to marry an elephant?' So strip off your loose clothes, take off your elasticated tights, corsets and orthopaedic body belts, and see the shape you're really in. Don't blame the mirror for what it reflects. What you see reflected from the glass is what you truly are – but is that how you want to be? Are you proud of what you see – the flabby arms, tubby tum and chubby cheeks? The actor Edward G. Robinson grew a beard in later life, telling his friends, 'It covers a multitude of chins.' But concealing your excess weight will do nothing to improve your health. So have a clear idea of how you'd like to look and then work towards that end. At fifty everyone has the body they deserve, for we are both the marble and the sculptor. So give yourself a visual target at which to aim. Find the most attractive picture you have of yourself taken before you put on weight and pin it to the mirror. If you had that kind of figure when you were young, there's no earthly reason why you shouldn't regain it over the next few months.

I've no time whatsoever for the American organizations which have been set up recently to fight against weight-based discrimination. They describe themselves as civil rights movements, but while they're right in describing obesity as a disability, it's a handicap which, unlike hemiplegia or congenital blindness, is self-induced and should never be made socially acceptable. Millions are spent on beauty products and cosmetic surgery, which shows that our personal appearance is one of the things that does most to give us a sense of justifiable pride. A recent study of a group of over three hundred women, aged between 18–65, attending British universities, revealed that nearly eight in ten would like to lose weight, with about a third claiming that they'd trade in a year of their life in exchange for a shapelier figure. The EssVee programme will achieve this end in just nine months. In this world there's no doubt that appearance matters. For a start, a shapely figure makes it easier to get a well-paid job, as will be described in the final chapter of this book. A pretty waitress receives five per cent more tips than her less attractive counterparts, and a retrospective study of the 1974 Canadian elections showed that good-looking candidates polled more than twice as many votes as less attractive nominees. These distinctions are even more apparent in the field of sexual attraction. Lonely hearts ads invariably invite replies from mates who are described as 'handsome', 'attractive' and 'slim', and frequently end with the request: 'photo essential'. One writer, seeking material for a feature about computer dating, reported: 'All the women I met or corresponded with rated physical attributes higher than personality traits – most of them believing relationships would stand or fall on physical attraction exclusively.' The same applies to the assessments we make when we're shown a series of portrait photographs. When we judge the people to be attractive, we automatically assume that they're also more sensitive, kind, interesting, sociable and sexually warm than those who are less good looking – a spill-over known as the 'halo effect'.

So don't place too much store on average height and weight tables, or measurements of your weight and BMI. Judge yourself by the way you look. Over the years I've noted that nudists are rarely fat. This may because they're already following an active, outdoor lifestyle, but I fancy they also take extra pride in their appearance since their bodies are constantly on show. Maybe that's why we call nude bathing 'skinny dipping' (I speak with some authority since I was once the European editor of two American naturist magazines). So view yourself from time to time in a full-length mirror and see what that impartial arbiter has to say. Maybe your weight hasn't so much risen as dropped, giving you an unattractive pear shaped figure. (Clothes shops now advise their checkout staff to look out for women who try to switch sizes on two-piece outfits. One stopped a woman who tried to do this with a pair of pyjamas and said: 'Madam you have a small top and a large bottom.' To which the indignant customer replied: 'You don't look so good yourself.') Keep a regular check on your physical appearance, and you'll lose weight, boost your self-esteem, improve your general health and physical fitness and gain the spin-off benefits of the 'halo effect'. But don't look too far ahead. Just focus on carrying out each week's assignment in the sure knowledge that once that's grooved you'll be one step nearer to your goal. Success will breed success.

> **STEP 3**
> Use a bathroom mirror to get a frank assessment of your present state, help you monitor your progress, and boost your pride and self-esteem, as you follow each step of the EssVee programme.

STEP 4

Hunger: the Finest Sauce and the Surest Guide to Calorie Intake

Animals in the wild are never fat. That's because Nature has provided them with an in-built mechanism which keeps them slim and maintains an automatic balance between their energy needs and their calorie intake. We have the identical homeostatic system, so why doesn't it work for us with equal efficiency? The answer is that it would, if we gave it half a chance. The problem lies in our evolutionary history, as has already been explained. We have inherited a propensity for storing fat, a tendency which is now bred into our genes. At one time this served a vital, life-preserving function. Now its mass effect is detrimental. Today it works to our disadvantage, making us prone to premature disability and decay, for we now live in an age of plenty, where our major hazard is not a dearth of food, but an unhealthy surfeit.

Surrounded by so many tempting foods, the truly amazing thing is not that we acquire a middle-age spread, but that by that time we're not all grotesquely obese. The average woman eats about twenty tons of food between the ages of twenty-five and sixty-five. During that time she gains an average of only twenty-four pounds of excess flab. That's a truly outstanding balancing act, for it represents an excessive intake of only an ounce of superfluous food a day. Nowadays we live in a world where we're encouraged to become food junkies, with the well-funded food companies acting as legally permitted pushers. The art of the confectioner, and the sole objective of the advertising industry, is to get us to eat more than we really need. How can we resist those enticing TV advertisements for chocolate layer cake? They're a mouth-watering invitation to over-indulge, with each two-inch slice supplying four hundred and fifty calories, which is nearly a fifth of the daily energy requirement of a sedentary female worker. Taken as an isolated indiscretion this may seem a mere trifle, but those extra calories are more than we need to put on a massive forty pounds of superfluous flab a year.

The fact that we don't suffer this fate is living testimony to the efficacy of the body's powers of self-regulation. Every mammal, whether it's a mouse, rat, dog, monkey or human being, is equipped with a weight regulating mechanism. We've chosen to call this closed-loop cybernetic system an 'appestat', since it works in exactly the same way as the thermostat which maintains the steady temperature of a central-heated house or office building. Experiments show that if the appestats of laboratory animals are destroyed, the animals overeat and become obese. Conversely, if they remain intact and are working normally, the creatures can be given unlimited quantities of food, and will only eat enough to balance their exact energy requirements. Given this inbuilt homeostatic mechanism, why do we come across so many overweight human beings? We shouldn't need to count calories, take slimming pills or submit to operations to reduce the size of our stomachs. All we need to do is pay attention to the wisdom of our bodies and eat solely in response to hunger cues.

There's a vast difference between hunger and appetite. Appetite is the *desire* to eat; hunger is the *need* to eat. Many people in the Third World are dying from a lack of nourishment, while those in the affluent countries are facing premature death from a surfeit of food. Our obesity pandemic could be stopped in its tracks if only we all agreed to follow the promptings of our appestats, and eat only when we're genuinely hungry. At present, most of us live in a state of perpetual satiation. Many adults, throughout their entire lives, have never experienced genuine hunger. This means they've never known the joy of sitting down to a meal when their mouth is watering and their stomach's registering the hunger pangs of eager expectation. Dionysius the Tyrant

21

was a glutton, and once complained that he wasn't enjoying the black broth that he'd been served. To this his head cook, braving a possible beheading, replied: 'I do not wonder, for the seasoning is wanted.' 'What seasoning?' his master replied. 'Running, sweating, fatigue, hunger and thirst; these are the ingredients with which we season all our food.' This truism was well expressed by a famous French chef who said: 'Hunger is the best sauce.'

Over time, you can solve your weight problem by doing nothing more than eating only when you're truly hungry. One lady followed this practice and over two years lost a vast amount of surplus weight. Having established the habit she felt confident that she wouldn't gain the weight she'd lost. So she put an advertisement in the local paper: 'Lost, three and half stone! Selling my fat clothes – good condition, sizes 18–20.' Over the next few days she was bombarded with phone calls. Nobody wanted to buy her discarded wardrobe – everyone was desperate to know how she'd lost the three and a half stone! The same practice helped Greta Garbo maintain her sylphlike figure. She refused to eat out of boredom or routine, and caused considerable amusement when she replied to a dinner invitation by saying: 'How do I know I'll be hungry on Wednesday?'

> **STEP 4**
> From now onwards learn to trust the wisdom of your body. Listen to the promptings of your appestat, and refrain from eating unless you're truly hungry.

STEP 5

Walking: The Perfect Tonic for Body, Mind and Spirit

Obesity is less often caused by gluttony than by sloth. Studies have shown that a number of overweight people actually eat less than average, and put on weight simply because they get too little exercise. This was confirmed when a study was made of the walking habits of a group of British volunteers, over half of whom were overweight. The results showed that, irrespective of the food they ate, the overweight subjects walked forty-two per cent less than those who retained their slim, youthful figures. To the researchers it seemed clear that it was the extra daily exercise that helped to prevent them developing a middle-age spread. Many people are put off when they learn that it's necessary to walk for nearly twelve hours to shed a single pound in weight. But nobody suggests that this trek has to be taken in a single day. We're aiming for long-term results, which means it can be spread out over a month or more. A middle-age spread will develop if you eat fifty calories a day more than you need to meet your calorie requirements. That's the equivalent of just ten minutes extra walking a day. Taking that small amount of additional daily exercise will shape, not only our ends, but also our middles.

This was demonstrated in convincing fashion when a sample of overweight patients was given the option of slimming by walking, or calorie-controlled dieting. Whatever choice they made, their routines were carefully controlled, so that the marchers burnt up five hundred calories more, while the dieters ate five hundred calories less. At the end of the sixteen-week trial period there was found to be little difference in the poundage the two groups had shed, but there was a marked difference in the distribution of that weight loss. The dieters had lost fat, but they'd also lost two and a half pounds of healthy muscle tissue, which left them feeling a trifle weak and wan. The walkers, on the other hand, had lost even more fat, but had also acquired one and a half pounds of solid muscle tissue, which made their bodies not only trimmer, but also firmer and stronger. Similar results were obtained in a trial carried out at the University of California's Metabolic Research Laboratory. In this experiment a group of overweight women were invited to eat whatever they liked provided they went for a daily walk of gradually increasing length. On this simple regime every woman became slimmer, and maintained her weight loss for a year or more. The average loss was twenty-two pounds, although some of the more enthusiastic walkers, carried away by the excitement of the experiment, shed as much as thirty-eight pounds.

This approach to weight loss can be effective even in the toughest cases. One American lady weighed well over twenty stone. Ashamed of her condition, when she caught sight of herself in a shop window, she decided to pay a return visit to her favourite health resort, where she'd been before when her predicament was less severe. She started her stay by having a private session with the hydro's psychotherapist, who studied her lifestyle and immediate saw that she needed to be more active. 'What's your favourite form of exercise?' he asked. This was not what she expected, because she'd come to the resort to be consoled and pampered, as she had been in the past, not to work out in the gym. For a while she couldn't think of a single thing she enjoyed which was even remotely energetic. The only activity which gave her pleasure, she finally confessed, was shopping. Seizing on this small gleam of hope, the scheming shrink invited her to do a deal. To help her lose weight, he got her to promise to walk once round the perimeter of her shopping centre before she went inside and made a purchase. By following this simple measure she shed three and a half stones in five months. You

may find this difficult to believe, but the loss is easily

explained for she usually visited the centre four times a week, and the trip round the perimeter of the block was a mile and a half long.

Anyone who takes this amount of walking exercise will lose weight. They'll also gain a trolley load of other goodies. Some while ago a long-term study of nearly nine thousand British civil servants revealed that men who walk for twenty or more minutes a day on their journey to and from work are fifty per cent less likely to develop heart irregularities than those who travel by bus or car. Many people find that walking is also an excellent way of shaking off bouts of anxiety and depression. This was the remedy practised by the philosopher Bertrand Russell, who had no doubt that 'unhappy businessmen would increase their happiness more by walking six miles a day than by any other conceivable change of philosophy'. So don't be surprised if a brisk walk goes to your head and gives you a hiker's high. The taking of a daily constitutional can also stave off some off the mental changes associated with the ageing process. This was revealed when researchers at the University of Illinois invited volunteers with an average age of seventy-two to walk for an hour three times a week. As a result, they showed an improvement in memory, attention and powers of decision making. A more recent study, carried out at the Texas Health Presbyterian Hospital in Dallas, showed that women who walk for thirty to fifty minutes a day, three or four times a week, raise the blood flow to their brain by as much as fifteen per cent. This, it's suggested, could reduce the risk of Alzheimer's disease, by bringing extra nutrients to the brain and 'washing away' the debris which is thought to contribute to the instigation of the disease. All these perks, and they're just a footstep away.

This is something we must teach our children from the earliest possible age. Some while ago a New Jersey schoolmaster grew alarmed at the flabbiness of many of his pupils and started taking them on long cross-country hikes. Within two years they were significantly leaner and fitter, and he himself had shed an impressive seventy pounds. Soon afterwards I told this story to a friend's roly-poly couch potato son. At the time he was lolling on a sofa sending out an endless stream of text messages. I suggested that, for a change, he should get up and go for a brisk walk, saying: 'Why do you think God gave us two legs?' Without looking up from his mobile phone he said with an air of bored resignation: 'One for the clutch and one for the accelerator?'

STEP 5
From now onwards get into the habit of taking a brisk daily walk lasting at least twenty minutes.

STEP 6

East Breakfast Like a King

If your get-up-and-go has got-up-and-gone, here's a simple way of boosting your energy levels which will also help to keep you slim. Every morning, before you start out on your day's activities, find time to sit down to a nourishing breakfast which includes some form of protein and fat, rather than just a hasty cup of coffee and a bite of toast which is taken on the hoof as you rush off to work. During the night, you may have been starved of food for twelve hours. That's why the first meal of the day should be a true breakfast. (The Spanish call the first meal of the day *desayuno*, which means 'breaking the fast'.) Unfortunately, throughout the industrialized world, breakfast is falling foul of our increasingly frenetic lifestyles. A study of three thousand people, carried out by scientists at the Children's Hospital in Boston, Massachusetts, showed that obesity was a third to a half lower in subjects who ate a good breakfast every day. They also had a reduced risk of developing 'insulin resistance', a biochemical aberration which predisposes to late onset diabetes. This was confirmed when researchers at the University of Tasmania tracked more than two thousand volunteers for a period of over twenty years. At the end of the trial it was found that starting the day on an empty stomach predisposes to obesity, larger fat stores around the belly, and higher cholesterol levels, three factors which are all markers for later heart disease.

For years we've been led to believe that eggs and bacon are bad for our health because of their high cholesterol levels. Now we're being reliably informed that we'd be healthier if they formed a regular part of our early morning meal. A recent study, carried out at the University of Alabama, compared two groups of mice. One was given a breakfast rich in carbohydrates, the other one which included generous helpings of fat. The results showed that the animals eating the cereals, croissants and rolls were more likely to gain weight, accumulate fat deposits, and develop signs of glucose intolerance, than the others. These are symptoms of the 'metabolic syndrome', which is associated with the development of heart disease and late onset diabetes.

At present, thirteen per cent of Britons confess that they're too busy to stop for a decent breakfast, which they recognize can make them tired and irritable. Equally disturbing, a recent survey of girls attending British schools revealed that nearly a third of fourteen- to fifteen-year-old girls admitted that they skipped breakfast in the misguided belief that this would help them lose weight. In fact the reverse is invariably the case, for studies have shown that three-quarters of the teenage girls who go without breakfast are overweight. This is probably because a mid-morning fall in blood sugar levels drives them to take calorie-rich snacks of biscuits and chocolate bars to boost their flagging energies. Skipping breakfast, as well as making us feel sluggish, also impairs our concentration. This is not surprising, for our mental functions always decline when our blood sugar levels fall. To keep cheerful throughout the morning, we also need to provide our brains with a generous supply of serotonin. This is a mood elevating neurotransmitter, derived from the amino acid tryptophan, which is found in protein-rich foods like oats, milk, eggs, red meat, yoghurt, fish, poultry and cottage cheese, which were once a standard component of the traditional English breakfast.

The first meal of the day varies widely around the globe. The Scottish have traditionally favoured porridge and kippers. In Nigeria it's customary to eat ogi, a porridge made from corn. Many Asian people start the day with a nourishing soup, made from meat, beans or lentils, sometimes topped up with leftovers from yesterday's meal. But time is short throughout the world, so short cuts are being made.

The Chinese have taken to eating a variety of dim sum dishes which they can buy in advance in the supermarket and quickly warm up in the microwave. And some Australians now fortify themselves with an equally speedily prepared smoothie called Up 'N' Go. But while eating patterns change, our nutritional needs remain the same. Whatever our nationality, if we eat an inadequate breakfast we increase our risk of becoming obese.

It may be no more than a coincidence, but the obesity epidemic started to rise some fifty years ago. At that time half the British population ate a cooked breakfast every day. Now less than one per cent follows this practice. This is a tragedy, for the English breakfast was once one of the wonders of the world. J. B. Priestley in his book *The Edwardians* tells of English gentlemen sitting down to breakfasts served from sideboards groaning with cold meats, pressed beef, ham, tongue, steak, woodcock, grilled trout and ptarmigan. As Somerset Maugham joked: 'The only way to eat well in Britain is to have breakfast three times a day.' Two generations later time constraints have reduced this meal to a quick snack, often of commercial breakfast cereals. The more popular these products are, and the more heavily they're hyped, the less nutritious they tend to be. Puffed rice is five times as expensive as ordinary rice yet provides smaller amounts of most nutrients. Without their added vitamins, many packaged cereals are hardly more nutritious than the cartons they're packed in. They fatten, but do little to prevent malnutrition. Their health claims are so much pap, cackle and puff.

Breakfast should include proteins and complex carbohydrates, because these take a while to be digested and so help sustain energy levels throughout the course of the morning. Proteins – like eggs, bacon, sausage and milk – are valuable because they raise the body's metabolic rate, which gets the day off with a warming start. Many of these dishes can be prepared overnight, including sandwiches filled with ham or cheese. Better to get up a half-an-hour earlier, than to skimp breakfast. Winston Churchill enjoyed a breakfast of grouse

29

and caviar. Babe Ruth, the legendary American baseball player, began the day with a meal of porterhouse steak, four fried eggs and a large portion of French fried potatoes, washed down with a pot of coffee and a large tot of bourbon whiskey. Both men realized the importance of making the first meal of the day a true break-fast. To preserve our health we should observe the South Americans' maxim: 'Eat breakfast like a king, lunch like a princess and dinner like a pauper.'

> **STEP 6**
> Start each day with a sustaining breakfast rather than a hasty snack.

STEP 7

Small Plates
Make for Svelte Figures

Has anyone ever suggested that most of the foodstuffs you eat every day aren't fattening, and that even includes the French fries you love and the chocolate biscuits you can't stop munching? Suppose you need 2,500 calories a day to keep your body in energy balance. Everything you eat up to that point can't possibly make you fat. The love handles appear only when you exceed that limit. In the past you may have been a serial dieter. Maybe at the moment you're trying the Omnivores diet, which you've embarked on because you quickly regained every pound you lost by following the Astronaut diet, and before that the Hollywood diet. All these regimes fail because they're unbalanced, artificial and abysmally dull. They all overlook one crucial factor, that eating is meant to be fun. It's a pleasure to be enjoyed, rather than a process to be endured.

Deep down, everyone knows that you can't be fit and fat. If you're carrying twenty pounds of excess flab you'll probably expend fourteen per cent more energy heaving yourself from place to place. This will make you tired, and also subject your joints to needless strain. With the exception of long-distance swimmers, whose weight is borne by the water, it's true to say that fat folk fade fast. Athletes take practical advantage of this knowledge, choosing to run in the lightest possible footwear because they know that they can make a one per cent saving in energy for every three and a half ounces they pare from their shoes. So how do you get yourself in fighting trim? Some years ago a team of dieticians came up with a novel approach to calorie control. They estimated that the average patient who came to them for slimming advice was one-eighth overweight. So they suggested they should curb their energy intake by dividing their food into eight sections. Seven of those portions they could eat, the remainder had to be thrown away. The argument was that it was better for food to go to waste – than to go to waist. In practice this advice is hard to follow. If food has eye-appeal we want to eat it all, every last mouthful, if only as a tribute to the chef. Besides, many of us were trained as children to clean our plates. 'Waste not, want not,' was one of my parents' favourite maxims, when we were struggling to eat the last of our meals. We had to be grateful for our good fortune, by eating every morsel of food the good Lord gave us but for some reason denied to the children in the undeveloped countries. Being a good trencherman I generally found this edict easy to follow, even though I could never understand how finishing my cabbage would help the thousands of starving children in India and sub-Saharan Africa.

A far simpler and more effective way of controlling food intake is not to throw food away, but to serve it on a smaller plate. Then it's possible to lick the platter clean without imbibing an excess of calories. The effectiveness of this technique has recently been confirmed by a series of experiments carried out by Dr Brian Wansink, Professor of Consumer Behaviour at Cornell University. He offered movie-goers a free supply of popcorn in containers of various sizes, and found that they ate forty-five per cent more when the containers were large rather than of a standard, smaller size. This even applied when the popcorn was stale, when the subjects were still tempted to eat a third more from the larger containers. This phenomenon is now known as the 'portion size effect'. If you need to reduce your calorie intake, take advantage of this physiological tendency, and serve your food on a smaller plate, then there's less risk that your eyes will be bigger than your belly.

David Wallerstein, who became a director of McDonald's, took practical advantage of this behavioural quirk. He started out in the cinema business, and was well aware of the significance of portion size. He found: 'People did not want to buy two boxes of popcorn.' So he made the popcorn containers bigger. As he later recalled, the results of this simple expedient 'were astounding'. People ate much more, which made them thirsty. This encouraged them to join the queues for the cold drinks and ice creams that the usherettes had on offer when the house lights went up. This response is not limited to people eating in groups. It's not that our gastric juices are stimulated by the sight of other people eating, although this undoubtedly happens. This was confirmed when forty American undergraduate students were asked to help themselves to snacks while watching a Super Bowl game. Those who were offered the snacks out of a large bowl ate fifty per cent more than those who were offered the same snacks supplied in smaller bowls. The truth is that we're very bad at judging our energy intake. We rely on visual cues, rather than training ourselves to respond to the internal satiety cues provided by our trusty in-built appestat. This is a faulty habit which must be changed. If not, we run the risk of eating to excess as a result of allowing our nutritional intake to be determined by such irrelevancies as the amount of food we're given, and the amount we feel we should leave on the plate.

STEP 7
Be aware of the 'portion size' phenomenon, and eat your food from small plates and modestly sized containers.

STEP 8

Fill Your Gut
with 'Good' Bacteria

Our world today is filled with strange ironies and bizarre contradictions. A typical example is the opposing aims of two of our major industries: food production and health care. While commercial farmers are struggling to find the quickest and cheapest ways of making their animals fat, the medical profession is engaged in an equally urgent battle to find the simplest and surest way of keeping its patients slim. This is a battle which up until now the farmers seem to be winning. They're using three techniques to fatten their animals, each of which can be used in reverse to tackle the obesity plague. Two of these are well known and already in everyday use. The third is largely ignored, but demands recognition and inclusion in the EssVee programme of lifestyle change.

At one time farm animals were allowed to roam free to forage for their food. Then it was found that chickens, pigs and beef cattle could be fattened more quickly if their movements were curtailed and they were fed high-energy foodstuffs. Those are recognized as two of the major reasons why human beings become obese. Like battery hens, many people are suffering because they're getting too little exercise and far too much food. But a third technique has been employed by the big agribusinesses to fatten their cattle which has largely gone unnoticed. When animals are kept in close confinement they're liable to suffer outbreaks of infectious ailments. These can be counteracted by dosing them with antibiotics, which keeps them disease-free and also helps them put on weight. This is the great commercial advantage of antibiotic medication, for if you sterilize an animal's guts, you destroy its flora of intestinal bacteria which would otherwise take nourishment from its host. This applies with equal force to humans.

Bacteria, in the past, have always had an exceedingly bad press. They're something we're always setting out to kill, not realizing that human life couldn't exist without their collaboration. We think of ourselves as the chosen race, yet bacteria are the true lords of the universe. They were the first forms of life to appear on the earth about four billion years ago, which is about the same time as rocks began to form. Since then bacteria have flourished. They've never risked extinction, because they can flourish in the most extreme environmental conditions. They're at home in high-temperature thermal vents and can equally well exist in sub-zero temperatures, corrosive acids and radioactive waste. They exist in countless species and sub-species and form a large part of the earth's biomass. The earth currently houses nearly seventy billion human beings and a phenomenal five *nonillion* bacteria.

Only a homocentric bigot could believe that *Homo sapiens* is the pinnacle and *ne plus ultra* of Darwinian evolution. The world belongs to bacteria not to man, as was clearly recognized by the late, great American scientist Stephen Jay Gould, who wrote 'This is the "age of bacteria" – as it was in the beginning, is now and ever shall be.' They've been both our tyrants and humble servants for 500,000 years, yet we didn't know they existed until 17 September 1683. That was the landmark day when the Dutch scientist Antony van Leeuwenhoek scraped some plaque from his tooth and examined it under a primitive, home-made microscope. It was then he saw what no one before had ever seen, or even suspected. His mouth was filled with a host of living organisms, which he chose to call *animacules* or 'little animals'. In a state of health, each adult has ten times as many bacteria in their guts as they have cells in their entire body. These are absolutely essential for the maintenance of our health, since they aid the digestion and absorption of our food. They also break down toxins, which might otherwise predispose to cancer and other serious ailments, and play an

35

essential part in the creation of vital enzymes and certain members of the vitamin B group. What's more, the 'goodies' among their number crowd out the 'baddies', which might otherwise multiply and give rise to serious intestinal diseases. By their very existence they also help to keep us slim. To survive, they've got to obtain a regular supply of nourishment, and that they can only obtain from the food we eat. Experiments, carried out by a team of researchers at Washington University School of Medicine, revealed that mice stayed slim only if they had the right balance of gut bacteria. As the team leader, Professor Jeffrey Gordon, explained: 'We never dine alone: our microbes are able to sit at the dining room table together with us, to consume for their own purposes the nutrients that are available.'

The contribution they make is quite considerable, and mimics the effect produced when our bodies are infected with intestinal worms. The film star Audrey Hepburn swallowed a tapeworm to keep slim, a ploy which was copied by one of her most famous fans, Maria Callas. She too lost a considerable amount of weight after swallowing a tapeworm, which many thought caused her to lose control of her top notes. But tapeworms are relatively puny things, compared with the three or four pounds of bacteria that make their home in our intestinal tracts. Troubles arise if we fail to support this full complement of healthy bacteria. Some of these are destroyed by the non-steroidal anti-inflammatory drugs we take to ease our aches and pains. Others are killed when we dose ourselves with medically prescribed anti-biotics, which can't differentiate between the bad bacteria which inflame our tonsils and the kindly bacteria which line our guts. More are dispatched by the antibiotic residues lingering in the meats we eat, and in the chlorinated water we're often forced to drink.

The simplest way to maintain a healthy level of bacteria in the gut is to take regular helpings of live yoghurt. This our nomadic forebears were doing in 10,000 BC, so it's hardly rocket science, but it will help to keep you slim. This was shown when a team of Japanese scientists gave eighty-seven overweight volunteers two daily doses of fermented milk. Those who imbibed yoghurt cultures rich in the bacteria our bowels favour – lactic acid bacillus, Bifidobacteria and Lactobacillus gasseri – lost an average of over two pounds in twelve weeks. During that time the circumference of their hips and waists fell by an average of just over one and a half centimetres. This shows that we're not only what we eat, but also what's eating us.

> ### STEP 8
> Maintain a healthy level of intestinal bacteria by eating regular helpings of live yoghurt.

STEP 9

Taking the Rough with the Smooth

Few things date as quickly as yesterday's health craze. One minute the vogue is for jogging, the next for colonic irrigation, yoga or Transcendental Meditation. We embrace these fashions with eager anticipation, then toss them aside like discarded toffee papers when they fail to live up to our expectations. So it is with our dietary fads and fancies. One minute the vogue is for vitamins, the next for fish oils, redcurrant juice or antioxidants. Since there's been no change in our biochemistry in the intervening years, isn't there a lingering chance that a food ingredient which was judged to be good for us once, might not continue to be of significant benefit? That's the question we need to ask about the 1980s' rage for dietary fibre.

This vogue stemmed from the pioneering work of Dr Denis Burkitt, a leading member of Britain's Medical Research Council, who had a strange yen to compare the bowel motions of native Africans with those of English schoolboys. In the course of his studies he found that Ugandan villagers, eating a diet rich in fruits and cereals, produced an average of nearly five hundred grams of faeces a day, which passed through their bowels in roughly thirty-six hours. These stools were more than four times as heavy, and passed twice as quickly through the gut, as those produced by boys attending English public schools. Burkitt surmised that this explained the high incidence of constipation in the Western world, which at the time was often described as 'the white man's burden'. He felt the finding might also explain why people in the developed countries had an increased risk of developing bowel cancer, for the longer food lingers in the gut the longer the intestinal walls are exposed to dietary toxins and carcinogens. One further study helped to clinch this hypothesis.

When Africans first arrived in America they suffered remarkably little bowel disease. Subsequently, when they exchanged their traditional diet of maize, millet and beans for 'civilized' foodstuffs like white bread, sugar and jam, they faced a greater chance of developing bowel diseases such as diverticulitis, appendicitis and polyps. Dr Burkitt's ideas were publicized in a book *Taking the Rough with the Smooth*, which suggested that the addition of two tablespoonfuls of bran, or five ounces of wholemeal bread, to the typical Western diet would provide sufficient fibre to improve bowel function and help prevent disease. It also hinted that people would be less likely to accumulate excess weight if they adopted a roughage-enhanced diet.

These ideas were initially ignored by a high percentage of his colleagues, but twenty years later they were given an enormous boost by the Royal College of Physicians, which published a report saying: 'It seems likely that a diet in which sugars and starches are taken in natural fibre-rich form would contribute to the control of obesity by encouraging satiety at a lower level of energy intake, and to a lesser extent by increasing the amount of potential energy lost in the faeces.' That public statement was welcomed with open arms by Audrey Eyton, the editor and co-founder of *Slimming Magazine*, who quickly devised a diet and recipe book based on Burkitt's principles. This was published in 1982 as *The F-Plan Diet*, a book which was a publishing sensation, selling over two million copies in numerous foreign language editions. Anyone who followed her instructions, she promised, would: 'lose weight more quickly than ever before, because a larger proportion of the calories you consume will remain undigested'.

That book is little read today, yet its fundamental message remains of crucial importance. The roughage we get from the cellular walls of plants provides almost no energy or calories, yet it remains a vital part of a healthy diet. The evidence shows that diets rich in roughage are associated not only with a reduced risk of obesity, but also with a lessened liability to heart disease and late onset diabetes. A study, carried out by researchers at the University of Sheffield, has shown that women who have the highest intake of fibre cut their breast cancer risk by half. Other trials have revealed that diets rich in fibre help to reduce blood cholesterol levels. And a recent Italian investigation, carried out by paediatricians at Florence University, has had even more wide-reaching implications. The researchers compared the health records of Italian children with those of their counterparts living in a rural West African village. The results revealed that the African youngsters, living on high fibre diets, had less asthma, eczema and inflammatory bowel disease than those in Florence, who regularly ate convenience foods rich in sugar and fats but desperately lacking in fibre. The Africans remained slim, not simply because they exercised more, but also because their stools contained three times the level of 'short term' fatty acids, the lipids excreted when the bowels contain a high level of 'good' bacteria of the sort associated with diets containing generous quantities of vegetables and wholegrain cereals. These facts have circulated around the world, and yet recent surveys reveal that the average American adult still consumes less than half the ideal daily intake of fibre. And the position is even worse for the Coke and candy US youngsters, many of whom are getting only a fifth of their recommended daily intake of roughage.

The message seems clear. If you want to remain slim without constant dieting, and wish to reduce your risk of succumbing to the chronic diseases of Western civilization, set out at once to reduce your intake of high energy, processed food and step up your intake of fresh fruits, raw or lightly cooked vegetables, bran, brown rice and wholemeal bread. This will create a feeling of fullness and satiate any lust you may have for cookies, chocolate bars and other calorie-rich confections. It will also aid the excretion of fatty acids, and foster the growth of colonies of healthy bacteria within your intestine, which was the objective of last week's habit change.

> **STEP 9**
> Ensure an optimum intake of dietary fibre, by eating plenty of fresh fruits, raw or lightly cooked vegetables, bran, brown rice and wholemeal bread.

STEP 10

Develop a Gourmet's Delight in Eating

This book has been written for people who love to eat but hate to diet. We are pleasure-seeking animals. The same, of course, is true of every other animal species. No one who's ever fed a pet can possibly doubt that eating is one of life's greatest joys. Give a dog a bone and it will be happy. So too are cats, when they've had their final lick of a plateful of cream. Such is the pleasure we get from eating, that laboratory animals will walk across grids which give them painful electric shocks in order to get a food reward. More remarkable still are the findings of experiments carried out in the 1950s by psychologist Dr James Olds. He was carrying out experiments to determine the neurological changes which took place when animals moved from a state of sleep to one of wakefulness. Quite by chance, he noted some exceptional responses when he planted electrodes in the brains of laboratory rats, inserting the probes into a specific part of the limbic system now known as the nucleus accumbens. Delving further into this serendipitous discovery, he discovered that the animals went berserk if he gave them the chance of pressing a lever which directly stimulated this cluster of nerve cells. Once they'd learnt this trick, the rats would ignore all other needs and passing distractions and press the lever obsessively up to five thousand times an hour. It quickly became clear that this was because the stimulus gave them intense pleasure. Subsequent experiments have been carried out on mice, guinea pigs, hamsters, rabbits, dogs, cats, fish and then even on humans. All show the same ecstatic response following activation of the nucleus accumbens, which has now been dubbed 'the pleasure centre'.

That centre is activated, not only when we eat food, but also when we see food or merely think about food. This was revealed by the Russian scientist Ivan Pavlov, who showed that if dogs were fed immediately after he rang a bell, they would quickly learn to salivate and drool even though he no longer gave them a food reward. This is known as a 'conditioned response', a reaction that humans show whenever they see advertisements for tasty foods. This is one of the reasons why people overeat. In their yearning to stimulate their pleasure centres, they ignore the wise promptings of their appestats. They see or smell a doughnut and the lever is pressed. We get instant gratification from eating succulent food, but no immediate reward for getting slim. That's the dilemma that faces every member of the corpulent corps. They won't get any pleasure from not eating hamburgers, in fact they'll get far less. That's a truth we can't escape. We can live without heroin and other addictive drugs, but we can't live without food. Every moment of every day we're surrounded by temptation.

That's one of the main reasons why slimming regimes fail. They provide punishment rather than reward. Every intelligent animal responds more readily to the carrot than to the stick. How on earth can slimmers be tempted by programmes of calorie counting, chemical sweeteners, diuretic pills and starch-reduced rolls? Mark Twain gave eloquent expression to their plight when he said: 'The only way to keep your health is to eat what you don't want, drink what you don't like and do what you'd rather not.' Eleanor Roosevelt was determined to keep a check on her husband's expanding waistline, so employed a nutritionist at the White House who was instructed to serve only 'health' foods. In an attempt to meet this brief, the menus he designed were nutritious but famously unappetizing. As a result Martha Gellhorn, wife of Ernest Hemingway, made a point of eating a full meal before she attended a White House dinner.

But there is a pleasurable alternative. Just as sex is for fun as well as for procreation, so food is for enjoyment as well as for nutrition. The choice isn't between being either a glutton or an ascetic. There is a middle way. The only sensible option is to make a conscious effort to become a gourmet, aiming to get the fullest possible pleasure from your food. Go for quality rather than quantity. Tickle your taste buds with caviar rather than chips. Linger over slices of delicately marinated gravlax rather than gorge on lumps of heavily battered fried fish. The Greek gods lived on ambrosia, while the Jews looked forward to living in a land flowing with milk and honey. You deserve a similar reward. Make an effort to source the very finest foods. Devote time to its preparation and derive the maximum possible enjoyment from its consumption. Savour your food as oenophiles enjoy their wine. First they gaze at it, so they can appreciate its appearance and quality. Then they take a deep sniff to pick up the subtleties of its bouquet. After that, they take a mouthful, and work it gently round their palates so they can get a full awareness of its taste. Only then do they allow the wine to slip from their mouth and slide into their stomach. Food should receive a similar treatment, each mouthful being allowed to linger in our mouths so we can revel in its appearance, texture, aroma and taste. Why should we settle for a hurried life of hamburgers and Coke when we can afford the joys of filet mignon and Chateau Lafite? Set out from now onwards to make gourmet eating part of your habitual lifestyle, then you'll lose weight, and gain pleasure.

STEP 10
Become a gourmet. Don't eat more, but do eat better.

STEP 11

Slow Down: You Eat Too Fast

One thing we frequently forget when we bolt our food, is that our stomachs have no taste buds. That means that the moment we've swallowed a portion of succulent food, maybe a slice of smoked salmon or a chunk of tasty Caerphilly cheese, we can no longer enjoy its aroma and flavour. We live in an age of constant hustle and bustle, but that hectic pace should never apply to the rate at which we consume our food. If it does, we run the risk of becoming gluttons rather than gourmets. Food must be given time to make contact with the taste buds in the mouth, most of which are housed in the front, back and sides of the tongue. It's also important for the food to be properly masticated, since solid foods are virtually tasteless. To get the maximum pleasure from our food, we must work much harder than sniffer dogs, whose sense of smell is over a million times keener than ours. Archie Moore, the world light heavyweight boxing champion, amazed his fans when he shed three stone in order to get back to the light heavyweight limit. He explained that he'd learnt a trick from an Aborigine, who said the secret was to thoroughly chew your food, but never swallow it! Mercifully there's no need for you to adopt this Spartan tactic. Providing you take time to digest your food, you can have all the pleasure and none of the pain.

The stomach has no teeth, which means that the process of digestion is impaired if food is not properly masticated in the mouth. The Victorians talked about 'head digestion', and stressed that it was vital to chew every morsel of food before it was swallowed. Tests show that after two hours in the stomach, only the outer portion of a piece of meat is digested if it's swallowed whole. If, however, the lump is thoroughly broken up in the mouth before it's gulped down, the digestive enzymes can reach every fibre, with the result that after two hours in the stomach practically all the meat is properly digested. Anyone who establishes this habit of unhurried eating will significantly reduce their risk of unwanted weight gain. Researchers at Laiko General Hospital, Athens, recently took blood samples from a group of people who were asked to eat ice cream at different rates. They found that those who ate slowly generated higher concentrations of two of the hormones known to be associated with a feeling of fullness. However, it takes several minutes before these chemicals reach the brain's satiety centre, during which time a good trencherman can consume another thousand calories.

For our primeval ancestors, the ability to eat quickly had a survival value. Now it can be a cause of premature death. We can't afford to be gobblers, an expression which has an interesting pedigree since it comes from the Early English word *gobbe* meaning mouth, and gives rise to such words as gob, goblet and gobbledegook. Unfortunately, the gobbling habit can start at an early age. This was shown when a team of researchers from the University of Southern California placed an observer to watch the eating patterns of children in a school cafeteria. After observing them for a month, they found that fat children were significantly faster eaters than thin children. A similar study of a large group of Japanese adults revealed that subjects who ate quickly trebled their risk of being obese. So it's clearly not just the calorie content of the food we eat that matters, it's also the pace at which we eat that counts. What you must do in future is devote more time to the sybaritic delights of head digestion, for that will give your appestat time to tell you when you've had enough. This was shown when Professor Edmund Rolls, a senior nutritionist at Oxford University, gave volunteers samples of chicken to chew and found that after five minutes their appetites had dropped significantly, even though they hadn't swallowed the food.

To help you curb the shovelling habit, it can help to make

45

a habit of putting your knife and fork down between each mouthful of food, or even switching to holding the fork in your right hand and the knife in your left. (Some years ago two American ladies invented a fork designed to encourage people to eat more slowly. Every time the battery-powered fork was used it shone a red light for 99 seconds. Once that time had elapsed the light changed to green, to tell the user that it was now permissible to take another bite. It's perhaps not surprising that the patented device did not catch on.) Maybe a better way to encourage a more leisurely pace of eating, and induce the right frame of mind, is to revert to the old practice of saying a brief grace before each main meal, especially those you take with family and friends. This can be done whatever your religious beliefs, if you recite the humanist grace which is now said before meals at Newnham College, Cambridge. This is delivered in Latin, but when translated into English reads: 'For food in a hungry world, for companionship in a world of loneliness, for peace in an age of violence, we give thanks.'

STEP 11
Maximize the pleasure you get from eating by lingering over the process of head digestion.

STEP 12

Avoid the Lure of Heavily Processed Foods

Health advisors are always ill advised to tell people what they shouldn't do, for fear of triggering what Freud termed the 'counter will', which is the overwhelming urge to do whatever we're told is 'naughty'. This is a fault I'm desperately anxious to avoid, which is why I'm struggling now to find an acceptable way of suggesting that you should give a wide berth to heavily processed foods.

Health professionals rarely agree on the steps their patients should take to lose weight, but now there's almost universal agreement that they should take urgent steps to reduce their intake of fats, sugar and salt. These are sometimes known as the 'toxic trio', since they're known to predispose to fatal conditions like obesity, type 2 diabetes and cardiovascular disease. These terrible triplets have an atavistic appeal, for at some stage primitive man must have discovered that he could travel more lightly if he filled his belly with fatty foods, since fats contain twice as many calories per ounce as proteins and carbohydrates. He also learnt to seek foods that had a sweet taste, because he then avoided those which had gone rancid. Instead he chose fruits and berries which had fully ripened and therefore had their maximum content of energy-rich sugars. His yearning for salt was probably even stronger, and longer established, for every mammal including man arose from the sea. When they migrated to the land, these creatures desperately needed to discover a source of salt, which was not to be found in fresh water rivers, springs and wells. Hence the appeal of salty foods, and salt licks, which animals will still trek thousands of miles to reach.

It is the recognition of this primeval fondness for fat, salt and sugar which now governs the formulation of commercial foods. The prime objective of the food industry is not to grow food, but to cultivate its revenues. In a world where the bottom line reigns supreme, companies aim to serve the short-term interests of their shareholders, rather than the long-term interest of their customers. Dr David Kessler, the former head of the US Food and Drug Administration, has written a damning book, *The End of Overeating*, which exposes the marketing strategies used by the big food companies. With the help of insiders, who have been prepared to blow the gaffe, he has revealed how the industry has engineered 'hyperpalatable' foods, creating goodies that we can't resist because they contain an optimized blend of the toxic trio. Food is now being larded with high-fructose corn syrup, which is cheaper and six times sweeter than sugar, but has the great disadvantage that it doesn't break down in the body but is shunted directly to the liver, from where it is immediately transported to the body's fat stores. Meats are being mixed with tenderizers and put into massive mixers, which break them down into tiny particles so they melt in the mouth without the need for chewing. The whole objective is to bypass our appestats, eliminate the need for any form of 'head digestion', and hit as quickly as possible what trade insiders call the brain's 'bliss point'. They know that once we get that first rush of pleasure, we'll carry on eating long after we've satisfied our energy needs. This is openly admitted by Procter & Gamble, who promote their Pringles crisps with the slogan 'Once you pop, you can't stop'.

In Britain, the government-sponsored National Institute for Health and Clinical Excellence has issued a statement urging the public to avoid eating commercial foods rich in saturated fats, sugar and salt. Such public appeals have been made for several decades but appear to be falling on deaf ears, for in just under twenty years at the close of the twentieth century the US consumption of fast foods tripled. One way of breaking this addiction is to shun all foods that are heavily promoted. Researchers claim that if people only ate food which was advertised on television, they would consume twenty-five times more sugar and twenty times more fat than is healthy. If firms find it necessary to spend a king's ransom to get you to eat their foods, through sophisticated media advertising, they clearly recognize that you wouldn't do so without their persistent coercion.

A worldwide crusade should be launched to restore the habit of eating real food, rather than ersatz manufactured substitutes. Once upon a time we sat down to consume our food, and ate only at set meal times. Now we can eat pretzels, pancakes, doughnuts, hot dogs, hamburgers, pizzas and Chinese takeaways at any time of the day and night. Teenagers can go into a Starbucks after school and buy a Frappuccino, which may contain the equivalent of eighteen teaspoons of sugar and six scoops of ice cream. In supermarkets it's estimated that junk foods now occupy a third of all shelf space. Sales of these hyperpalatable foods represent the fastest growing segment of the food industry, and provide far higher profits than fresh fruit and vegetables, which deteriorate more quickly, have a smaller mark-up and occupy more shelf space. When you're running a public company your eyes must be focused on the bottom line. This means that the health of your balance sheet must always take precedence over the health of your customers. The same applies to the fast food eateries, which can do nothing to increase the size of their local populations, and so can only boost their profits by tempting each customer to eat a little more. This is why in the last half century the calories in a standard serving of McDonald's French fries have more than tripled. These eateries, and the supermarket shelves laden with junk foods, should be avoided like the plague they're causing.

STEP 12
Resolve to avoid eating hyperpalatable processed foods and rediscover the pleasure of eating real, fresh, organic foodstuffs.

STEP 13

Have a Good Night Out – at Home!

The step you took last week leaves a yawning gap which must be filled. If you stop eating junk food in fast food restaurants, where now do you take your meals and get your gastronomic pleasures? The obvious answer is to return to the age-old habit of preparing and eating food in your own home. This will not only improve your diet, but also go a long way toward solving one of the developed world's major social problems. For some years family life has been in sad decline in most industrialized countries. A survey carried out in 2010 for National Family Week revealed that one in eight UK families now spend no more than two hours a week as an integrated family unit. Surveys reveal that Americans now spend just under half of their food expenditure on eating out, which is practically twice the amount they spent fifty years ago. Rather than joining together around the family dining table – as the folk artist Norman Rockwell depicted in his famous painting *Saying Grace* – they now eat a Taco Cabana in their car, or phone for a delivery of a Burger King or Kentucky Fried Chicken. We live in a fragmented and frenetic world, where a pizza gets to your home quicker than the police or fire brigade.

We are, by nature and nurture, group animals. Communities are built up of family units, and if family life is allowed to crumble the whole fabric of society is thrown into disrepair. In the Middle Ages, even if families were separated during the working day they came together at night to eat and gather around the family hearth, and possibly even to sleep together in a communal household bed. In Victorian times the family unit was frequently larger, but every bit as close. Adults and children prayed together, took their share of the household chores and made their own entertainment, singing songs around the piano or playing endless games of Ludo, Snap and Happy Families. The advent of modern technology has sounded the death knell of this domestic accord. In the evenings we no longer cluster together around the living room fire. Central heating has made it possible for children to retire to their own rooms to watch television, play computer games or send text messages to their friends. Today we try to live convivial lives by proxy. We watch soap operas, tweet, and take part in internet chat rooms and forums. But cyberspace encounters can never compensate for real space contacts. Besides, these are sedentary activities which do little to burn up calories and boost our metabolic rate. True conviviality comes only when we live together, which is the very origin of the word *convivere*.

Microwave ovens, and takeaway meals, have enabled us to gobble our food when and where we want. We no longer need to eat *en famille*, unless we have the privilege of being the President of the USA. This is one of the perks of living in the White House, according to President Barack Obama who told a *Time* reporter: 'Among the many wonderful things about being President, the best is that I get to live above the office and see Michelle and the kids every day. We have dinner every night. It is the thing which sustains me.' Round the dinner table the family talk, and play 'thorns and roses', a game in which they recount the good and bad things that have happened to them during the day.

The more we eat out, the more calories we'll consume. This was revealed by an American study which followed the eating activities of three thousand young adults for fifteen years. The results showed that those who ate fast food more than twice a week gained nine to eleven pounds more weight than those who ate it once or less per week. If we eat at home we have to source our foodstuffs, prepare them for cooking, carry them from kitchen to dining table, then stack the dishes and probably wash the pots and pans. All these activities keep us on the move and help to burn calories. As an

51

added reward we'll be eating food which is invariably more nourishing and also far less likely to carry harmful germs. This has been confirmed by bacteriological studies which reveal that half of all disease outbreaks result from food prepared and bought outside the home.

Recent evidence suggests that while we're doing away with single-purpose dining rooms, we're becoming increasingly fond of dining in and home cooking. This is a habit which must be fostered. A British study, carried out in 2005, revealed that the proportion of family meals eaten at the table was thirty-six per cent higher than it was in the previous year. And a more recent survey, conducted by UK Meat & Livestock Commission, showed that the percentage of young women claiming that they 'enjoyed cooking' had risen by nearly eighty per cent. This was almost certainly due to the plethora of TV documentaries offering mouth-watering demonstrations of haute cuisine cooking. We can halve our overheads, and double our fun, if we share home-cooked meals with family, friends and neighbours. That is in accord with the old proverb: 'It is better to want meat, than guests or company.' Everyone enjoys meals to celebrate family birthdays and weddings, so why can't we have these funfests more often – like once a week? What's the best thing about Christmas? a group of people was asked when they'd just finished the last of their cold turkey and mince pies. Two per cent said the presents, three per cent the food, seven per cent having time off work, and a massive eighty-six per cent the joy of spending time with family and friends. This is something we should aim to enjoy as often as we can, for while bricks and mortar make a house, it's the laughter and companionship of family and friends that make a home.

STEP 13

Devote more time and attention to home cooking, increasing your enjoyment whenever possible by sharing your meals with family, friends and neighbours.

STEP 14

Harness Muscles to Improve Your Figure While You Sleep

Our bodies contain well over six hundred muscles. These make up forty-two per cent of the body weight of an average man, and thirty-six per cent of the mass of a typical woman. The influence they have is immense, for our skeletal muscles not only power our movements but also mould our figures and shape our posture. We put on weight only when our calorie intake exceeds our calorie output. One painless way of burning excess calories is to carry out exercises designed to produce a gentle increase in our muscular framework, for this consumes a high percentage of daily energy input. Weight for weight, even when they're at rest, our skeletal muscles consume nearly three times more energy than our fat stores. This means that the more muscles we maintain, the easier it becomes to stay slim. To emphasisze this point, it might help if this week you thought of obesity as a lack of muscle rather than a surfeit of fat

People who embark on a typical eight-week weight training programme normally gain from three to five pounds of solid muscle. This means that so long as they maintain that gain, they'll be burning up dozens of extra calories a day just by sitting still! The more muscle tissue we retain, the less we need to monitor our food intake. While glucose is being used up by our muscles, it can't be taken to the liver, converted into glycogen and then stored as fat. But once again it pays to make haste slowly. Ignore the fitness trainer's goading slogan 'No pain, no gain.' Take it gently. Build your body a step at a time. Try to spend fifteen minutes less each day in passive activities, like reading magazines and watching TV, and devote the time you've saved to a gentle and progressive course of body-building exercises.

This programme should be of your own choosing. I start the day with a schedule of sit-ups and press-ups, but you may prefer to go a gym, or make use of exercise devices like dumb-bells, chest expanders, rowing machines, treadmills and static bicycles. These will all build muscle bulk, providing you realize that what you get out of them is directly proportional to what you put in. There's no machine in the world that can strengthen your muscles without effort on your part. That was the promise of the old faradic machines, which promised that if you lay on your back with electrodes attached to your thighs, belly or buttocks you could tighten your torso in minutes, without the need to make the slightest exertion. This is an absolute myth. You'd get more exercise putting on a tight pair of jeans. At one time firms would advertise these devices with the promise: 'Within a week you'll have a firm waistline which will be the envy of your friends. Thirty day FREE TRIAL.' Now tell me, how can any company make money if you can get a flat stomach in a week, and have the course free for a month?

Most people as they age put on weight, and show a decline in their muscle bulk and strength. They don't grow *up* they grow *out*. But this is by no means inevitable. The decline is the product of disuse atrophy. We're living longer than ever before, but those extra years are a drag if we've lost our get-up-and-go. That's why medical statisticians today make a sharp distinction between 'active life expectancy' and 'dependent life expectancy'. The first is a blessing, the second a curse. The way to ensure that old age continues to 'burn and rave at close of day' is to keep fit. A forty-year study of nearly six thousand men, carried out by the Pacific Health Research Institute in Honolulu, revealed that grip strength was an accurate determinant of healthy longevity. This is an indication of upper body strength, and shows that 'better built organisms last longer'. Many old-stagers shelter behind the excuse that it's normal for muscles to turn to fat with the passage of time. In fact these changes are coincident rather than consequential. If we're idle, muscles waste at the same time as fat is accumulated, which gives the impression than flesh is turning to flab.

Whatever our age we must take steps to maintain our muscle mass. The best way to start is by strengthening the legs, which will improve our balance and decrease our risk of falls. It will also lessen our chance of developing osteoporosis, for when extra blood is driven to the muscles, it's also carried to the underlying bones. When students at the University of Illinois were given weight training exercises five times a week to strengthen their leg muscles they made rapid gains in both power and endurance. After ten weeks their muscles were forty to fifty per cent stronger and they took forty-seven per cent longer to reach the point of fatigue when tested on cycle ergometers. If improvements like this can be made with fit young men, just think of the benefits they'll provide for forty-year-olds, who for years have done nothing more strenuous than turning the ignition keys of their cars. Try to find some time every day to climb up and down a flight of stairs. (You'll use up three times as many calories going up as coming down.) Do a series of heel raises every time you brush your teeth, and a few semi-squats while you're waiting for the kettle to boil. These are best done by placing your hands on your hips and bending the knees until they're parallel to the ground. After holding that position for a brief while, return to the upright position bracing your knees backwards as tightly as possible to strengthen your quadricep muscles.

Muscle-building exercises can be done at any time and place. An excellent way to tone up the belly wall, for instance, is to perform an 'abdominal retraction', which means drawing in the tummy wall in an effort to pin the navel against the spinal column. This can be done at odd times during the day, while waiting for a bus, or standing in line in a checkout queue. In the same way, resistance exercises can be carried out while watching TV or sitting in a car. These are often called isometric exercises, because the muscles contract against resistance without any change in

55

their actual length. A simple example is clasping the hands together and alternatively pushing and pulling. This is a highly effective way of building muscle tissue, as was shown by a study carried out a few years ago at the East Carolina University which revealed that resistance exercise leads to more weight loss than jogging, squash and other forms of aerobic exercise. If we care for our muscular tissues, our muscles will work day and night to care for us, keeping our bodies shapely and trim and burning up the excess calories which would otherwise be deposited in our fat stores.

> **STEP 14**
> Set aside time every day to maintain the strength and bulk of your skeletal muscles.

STEP 15

In Praise of the Stone Age Diet

Most dietitians believe that our tendency to put on weight results from our adoption of a 'civilized' diet to which we're not yet attuned. They're convinced that our health would be enhanced if we reverted to a 'Stone Age Diet' rich in proteins, vegetables, nuts and fruit. Six weeks ago we recommended the adoption of a high roughage diet, now we're repeating that advice for a slightly different reason. The brain's satiety centre receives information from stretch receptors in the stomach, which lets it know the state of its distension. If the stomach is empty we may get the cue to eat. When it's full, it may tell us that we've had enough. Highly concentrated energy foods are slow to arouse these signals. A Big Mac weighs one hundred grams and supplies well over two hundred calories. The identical weight of cabbage provides just seventeen calories, which is a vast difference.

Our lives are totally dependent on the chlorophyll in green plants. Only these cells can trap the sun's rays and convert them into edible, carbohydrate foods. Most of the dinosaurs, which ruled the planet for millions of years, were total herbivores, sustaining their vast bodies with whatever plant foods they could scavenge. Fossil records reveal that it was only when these monsters were wiped out, that the earth's vegetation could flourish and support the growth of other creatures. With the disappearance of the dinosaurs, mammals increased in size from a maximum weight of about twenty-two pounds to an elephantine seventeen tons. Man was the major beneficiary of this green explosion.

For decades the term 'health foods' has been reserved for commercially manufactured products. Now it's beginning to be used to describe a wide variety of vegetables which

medical research has shown to have some remarkable therapeutic properties. On a green diet we lose weight and gain a
wide range of other health benefits. This was demonstrated
some years ago when twenty healthy volunteers were put on
a Stone Age Diet for three weeks. At the end of this time a
check-up revealed that they'd lost an average of roughly five
pounds in weight, and reduced their waist measurement by
one and a half inches. Despite this evidence, and massive
government-funded advertising campaigns, only a mere nine
per cent of Americans today are getting their recommended
daily ration of five portions of fruit and vegetables.

When researchers at Stanford University, California, took
a sample of over a hundred adults with mildly raised cholesterol levels, they found that those who were encouraged to
step up their intake of fresh fruits and vegetables enjoyed a
reduction in their 'bad' cholesterol levels which was twice
that of those who'd followed the typical instructions to
reduce their intake of fatty foods. Another study, carried out
at Exeter University, showed that athletes who drink a glass
of beetroot juice every day increased their stamina by twelve
per cent. There's also been good news from the University
of Wageningen in the Netherlands, which demonstrates that
people aged fifty to seventy have the mental ability of
subjects five years their junior if they eat a diet rich in folic
acid, a naturally occurring nutrient found in broccoli,
Brussels sprouts, peas, chickpeas and fruits like oranges and
bananas.

One needs a degree in nutritional science to understand
the minutiae of these exciting discoveries. But we can
recognize the general drift and extract their practical
benefits, by going native and eating the widest possible
variety of berries, fruits and vegetables, each of which
contains its own range of health-giving antioxidants,
enzymes and micro-nutrients. Research on mice, carried out
at the Texas Women's Hospital, reveals that the polyphenol
antioxidants in blueberries can cut the number of fat cells in
the body by almost three-quarters, and smaller doses by
more than a quarter. A similar study of eighty middle-aged

women, conducted by scientists at Florida University, showed that subjects who ate 75 grams of apple a day for six months lost an average of over three pounds in weight, coupled with a reduction of nearly a quarter in their blood levels of 'bad' cholesterol. This suggests that an apple a day may well keep the doctor at bay, and maybe the mortician as well. Other investigations on laboratory mice, undertaken at the University of Western Ontario, Canada, revealed that many citrus fruits contain a flavonoid called naringenin, which causes the liver to burn fat rather than send it to the body's fat stores. Since it's difficult to keep up with the findings of this exciting research work, we need to hedge our bets by eating the widest possible range of fruit and vegetables.

A short while ago a Frenchman, paying his first visit to England, said: 'The English have only three vegetables – cabbage, cabbage, cabbage.' Mercifully that mindset is beginning to change but people in all the developed countries must become more adventurous, copying the example of the Kalahari bushmen, who include about seventy different vegetables in their routine diet. History shows that we're always healthier when our diet is rich in fresh fruit and vegetables. It's commonly thought that the nutritional standards, and life expectancy, of working-class families was appalling at the start of the twentieth century. In fact they were infinitely better fed than the average person today. Rural workers lived on readily available local food, which meant that they were generally well nourished and capable of carrying out heavy manual work. Estimates suggest that they consumed about ten portions of fruit and vegetables a day, which is at least three times more than the average person eats today. Because of their nourishing diet and healthy, outdoor lifestyle they were ninety per cent less likely to succumb to the killer diseases which afflict us today, such as obesity, cancer, heart disease and type 2 diabetes. Nutritional problems only arose with the advent of the Industrial Age, when people migrated into the cities, took less exercise, and began to eat more canned and processed foods rather than their traditional country fare. As a result, half of the British men who volunteered to fight in the Boer War were rejected because they lacked the required level of physical fitness. To boost our health, and whittle our waists, we need to return to the diet that sustained the health of our Stone Age forebears.

STEP 15
Expand your diet to include the widest possible range of fresh fruits and vegetables, and you'll become both lighter and better nourished.

STEP 16

Come Alive. Switch On. Enjoy!

Babies hate to be taken from their mother's breast. When they become toddlers, they're equally peeved if you stop them eating a lollipop. So it is for adults, if you reduce their overdraft limit, or take away their grown-up toys. As a species, the human race is averse to any form of deprivation. Psychologically, we invariably find it more appealing to take things up, than give them up. That's one of the main reasons why dieting fails. What we need is a change of lifestyle, which replaces passivity with spirited activity. Instead of focusing on the depressing chore of calorie-counting dieting, we should set out to adopt a more dynamogenic way of life. Then, while we're having fun, our metabolic fires will burn more fiercely and consume any surplus calories we might have consumed.

A team of psychological researchers at the New England Medical Centre studied the personalities of a mixed bag of over two hundred women, some of whom were fat and some slim. The results revealed that the chance of becoming over-weight is partly determined by our underlying character traits. The chubby ladies in the survey were found to be more repressed, and more given to daydreaming, than those of normal weight. As a group they showed more tension and anxiety. When they were in a tight corner, they tended to turn their anger and frustration inward upon themselves, rather than express it outwardly. Preoccupied with their own concerns, they showed little interest in others, retreating into what the researchers dubbed their 'fortress of fat'. In this introspective state, they derived their satisfaction from feeding their face, rather than nourishing their relationship with their family and friends. The slim subjects, on the other hand, obtained their pleasure, not from self-indulgence, but through their constant interaction with other people and the world around them. By disposition, they were vivacious and outward going. They lived *con brio*, a musical term for showing spirit, verve and energy. This is a life-affirming disposition, which can be acquired, by steady practice.

Dr James Levine and a team of researchers from the Mayo Clinic, Minnesota, took a group of twenty sedentary workers and divided them into two groups. Half were lean, the others mildly overweight. For ten consecutive days the subjects' activities were monitored, using movement sensors embedded in their underclothes which registered their slightest twitch. The results showed that small, but sustained, changes in daily living can have a profound effect on a person's weight and overall energy balance. Even chewing gum uses about eleven calories an hour, which is twenty per cent more than a person consumes when they're totally at rest. Doing the ironing consumes a hundred and forty calories an hour, and other household activities like vacuuming considerably more. A serious kiss burns six calories, and a session of lovemaking fifty times as much. Women who knit while they're watching TV burn up an extra twenty calories an hour. If they did this every day they'd be at least two pounds lighter by the end of a year. More energy would be consumed if they sat in a rocking chair and spent three hours an evening rocking gently to and fro. This will burn up an extra fourteen thousand calories, which is equivalent to a loss of four pounds of fat a year. Anyone who combines enough of these extra, micro-activities will show a slow, but inexorable, decline in their body weight.

Couch potatoes put on weight because they spend too long sitting down. According to Dr Levine, obese people sit an average of one hundred and fifty minutes more each day than their lean counterparts. As a result they burn three hundred and fifty fewer calories a day, which represents a weight gain equivalent to thirty-three pounds a year. On the basis of these findings, Dr Levine wants schools to strip their classrooms of chairs. This one measure alone, he thinks, would help keep youngsters slim. To test this theory, he carried out a week-long experiment in Britain, in which he got teachers to give their lessons in specially adapted classrooms. Instead of sitting at traditional desks, the volunteer class of children used 'lean and move' tables where they could work while standing up. (Floor cushions were provided should they need to take a rest.) As a result, the youngsters spent an average of five hours a day standing, a posture that burns up three times more calories than sitting. 'From our early findings,' reports Dr Levine, 'I would say that this approach has the potential to prevent an obesity epidemic in children.' Adults should adopt the same practice whenever they can. Anyone who spends three-quarters of an hour a day on the telephone could burn up about a pound of unwanted fat a year simply by refusing to be chair bound when they take their calls.

This switch will be beneficial, not only for your figure, but also for your general vitality and overall health. Some years ago five healthy volunteers in their late twenties agreed to stay in bed for three weeks. At the end of that brief spell of enforced idleness, doctors found that their muscle power had dropped, which led to a twenty-six per cent fall in their cardiac output and a thirty per cent decline in their respiratory capacity. According to the researchers, these changes meant that the young men had aged thirty years in just three weeks! Most of the drugs that have been prescribed to help people lose weight – such as amphetamine and thyroxine – have proved effective because they've increased the level of people's metabolic activity. Tranquillizers have the opposite effect. In December 2006 the American press published leaked documents, obtained from the drug company Eli Lilly, which revealed that one-third of patients taking the firm's anti-depressant drug Zyprexa for a year had gained at least twenty-two pounds, with half of them showing a massive hike of over sixty-six pounds. *New Scientist* magazine, commenting on these figures, said that drugs like these which slow us down, 'could potentially be causing a significant – and growing portion of America's obesity problem'.

To tackle our contemporary woes we need, not drugs, but the adoption and pursuit of a healthy way of life. Obesity can be overcome by embracing a dynamogenic lifestyle, a modus vivendi in which our days are filled with excitement, vitality, laughter, love and the joyful company of lively friends. This is the 'Live-More-Weigh Less' regime, an approach which, if you adopt it, will add life to your years and years to your life.

STEP 16
Increase the tempo of your life,
and learn to live with spirit and verve.

STEP 17

The Nibbler's Diet

Everyone knows that strenuous activity – like weightlifting, hill climbing and playing squash – acts as a powerful metabolic stimulus. But how many people realize that the mere fact of eating boosts the body's metabolic rate by twenty to thirty per cent? This basic physiological fact is one of the open sesames to safe and simple slimming. If you want to maintain a sylphlike figure without effort or fuss, it's a big mistake to follow the Western custom of existing on one or two large meals a day. A far better practice is to copy the Oriental example and spread your food intake over a series of small snacks, taken whenever you feel a trifle peckish. Anyone who visits Malaysia or Thailand for the first time will be struck by the sight of roadside vendors catering for this particular need. From dawn to dusk, they'll be serving a wide variety of snacks made from noodles, beans, sweet potatoes and rice porridge. In this way they enable the locals to satisfy their energy needs without feeling either hungry or over-full. Most Westerners who've adopted this eating pattern have lost weight.

The film star Marlon Brando battled with weight problems after his worldwide success in *A Streetcar Named Desire*. After appearing in *Sayonara*, his co-star and lover, the Oriental beauty Miko Taka, persuaded him to adopt the Nibbler's diet. Instead of tucking into one or two major meals, she persuaded him to eat eight snacks a day. These generally consisted of banana sandwiches and a glass of his favourite coconut milk. On this regime he quickly lost ten pounds, which he soon regained when he reverted to his old ways. A better example is Kim Dudley, a rotund middle-aged accountant who was known to his colleagues as 'Cuddly

Dudley'. His problems arose because he'd acquired the habit of keeping himself going throughout his stressful working days by drinking heavily sweetened cups of coffee, supplemented from time to time with biscuits and Mars bars. In a vain attempt at girth control he'd tried a number of weight reducing diets, and made several visits to health farms. But every attempt to slim was foiled by the fact that he loved to eat and felt miserable and faint the moment he stopped. In desperation, he sought the advice of his doctor, who suggested he should adopt a nutritious Nibbler's diet. This regimen worked like a charm and was the easiest 'diet' he'd ever followed. Within ten weeks he shed just over a stone. At this point his colleagues stopped calling him Cuddly Dudley, and promised that if he followed the treatment for another few months they'd switch to calling him 'Tiny Tim'.

These anecdotal case histories are now backed by a wealth of medical research. Several years ago a trial was carried out at Michael Reese Hospital, Chicago, in which a large colony of rats was divided into two identical groups. All the animals received the same allotment of food. One group was forced to consume their calories in two set meals, while the others were allowed to nibble their rations whenever the fancy took them. At the end of the forty-one day test period the rats were weighed, and it was found that the ones existing on the two set meals had accumulated twice as much fat as the grazers. Subsequent autopsy studies have shown that when rats are given heavy meals, their stomachs and small intestines expand by an average of forty per cent. This aggravates their weight problem, because they now have a greater surface area to absorb their intake of fats and sugars.

Similar studies have now been carried out on humans. Workers at the Institute for Clinical and Experimental Medicine in Prague have investigated the eating habits of a group of well over five hundred adult males. At the start of the project they discovered that the men were accustomed to eat anything from one to six meals a day. When biochemical tests were taken, it was found that those who were in the habit of consuming five or six meals a day were lighter, carried less body fat and had significantly lower blood cholesterol levels than those who ate three or fewer meals a day. A similar study was carried out by Toronto researchers, who followed a group of volunteers for four weeks. During the first two weeks the men were instructed to eat their food in three set meals – breakfast, lunch and dinner. For the final fortnight they ate exactly the same food, but this time as *seventeen* small snacks. Blood studies revealed that when they were on the second diet, their blood cholesterol levels were over eight per cent lower. This was accompanied by a fall of fifteen per cent in their lipoprotein levels and a twenty-eight per cent reduction in their mean insulin levels. This meant they were less likely to put on weight, and carried a reduced risk of getting both heart disease and type 2 diabetes.

For the sake of your life line, as well as your waist line, there seems little doubt that you'd be better off as a grazer than a *fresser*, a lovely Yiddish word derived from the German *fress* meaning 'devour'. So set out from now onwards to ape the Oriental races by switching to a Nibbler's diet. This involves having a modest breakfast, lunch and evening meal, supplemented by snacks in the mid-morning and mid-afternoon. These mini-meals can consist of a bowl of thick soup; a slice of wholemeal bread and a portion of cheese; a banana; a glass of milk; a small handful of nuts and raisins; a cupful of muesli, or a helping of yoghurt. On this regime, providing you don't increase your overall intake of calories, you'll find you'll start to lose weight without feeling hungry. The long-term aim is to eat like a bird – providing it isn't a vulture!

STEP 17
Instead of limiting your food intake to one or two large meals, adopt the habit of eating five or six small snacks per day.

STEP 18

Soup of the Day

Soups, broths and potages are the oldest recorded cooked foods, archaeologists having unearthed evidence which shows they date back over eight thousand years. Once early man had mastered the art of creating hearths and lighting fires, he quickly found that broths offered an excellent way of extracting the full food value of vegetable scraps and animal carcases. When permanent homesteads were established their appeal continued, because they provided a tasty, nourishing dish which even the poorest families could afford. In sixteenth-century France, cheap, but invigorating, soups were sold by street vendors who offered them as a remedy for physical exhaustion. These dishes became so popular among the working classes that in 1765 a Parisian entrepreneur decided to take them upmarket and offer them in well-furnished indoor eateries. These establishments came to be known as 'restaurants', since they were places specializing in the provision of 'restoring' food. In this way they served the same function as the Oriental street vendors mentioned in last week's assignment.

Starting a meal with a bowl of soup is an excellent way of keeping slim. This was demonstrated by researchers at Pennsylvania State University, who gave volunteers a lunch which either went straight to the main course, or started with a consommé or broth soup. Both of these soups were made from the identical ingredients: chicken broth, broccoli, potato, cauliflower, carrots and butter. The results were unambiguous. Those who started with the soup, whether it was thick or thin, received a high intake of fluid and roughage which quelled their hunger pangs and gave them a feeling of satiety. As a result they consumed an average of twenty per cent fewer calories when they finally tucked into their main course. 'People on diets are usually restricting their food intake, which is not always effective because they feel they are missing out on eating,' the researchers explained. 'What our study shows is that when volunteers had soup they were eating more food but consuming fewer calories.'

Eating some soups can also have a therapeutic effect, which is why chicken soup became exceedingly popular among Jewish families living in straitened circumstances in the European ghettoes. Its effect is partly sedative, which is why Jack Canfield and Mark Hansen chose to call their collection of inspirational stories *Chicken Soup for the Soul*, a book which went on to sell in excess of two million copies. Now I was once a great fan of chicken meat, because it originally contained so much less fat than Aberdeen steaks. But that's only true of free-range chickens fed on a natural diet. Corn-fed battery birds are a totally different species. This was revealed by a trial carried out at the London Metropolitan University, which showed that, as a result of the radical change in farming methods, chicken meat now contains nearly three times as much fat as it did thirty-five years ago. A roast chicken leg complete with skin now has more fat than a Big Mac. 'Chickens used to roam free and eat herbs and seeds,' the researchers explained. 'They are now fed with high energy foods and even most organic chickens don't have to walk any distance to eat.'

So we may have to revise some of our ideas about chicken soup, although the evidence suggests that it can still have a calming effect on the mind, because it's one of the finest sources of tryptophan, the precursor of serotonin, a naturally produced hormone which lowers levels of aggression, encourages restful sleep and generates a stable mood and equable temperament. This is classified as an 'essential' amino acid because it can't be produced in the body, but must be obtained through the diet. But the great joy of soup is that it can be made from whatever scraps of meat and vegetables happen to be around. It offers a dish which is not only delightfully varied, but also provides a wide range of minerals, vitamins and other essential nutrients. In the Ukraine it's made with beetroot (Borscht); in the south of France from scraps of fish (Bouillabaisse); in Scotland from leek and potatoes (Cock-a-leekie) and in Italy from mixed vegetables (Minestrone). For a brief while in England it was fashionable for the landed gentry to sit down to Green Turtle Soup, made from giant turtles, weighing up to a hundred pounds, which were shipped over live from the West Indies in fresh water tanks. Within weeks of their grand display on the tables of the trendsetting moneyed classes, inventive traders were offering the hoi polloi the chance to follow the fashion by eating 'mock' turtle soup made from the heads of wild boars.

Whether your taste is for bisques or broths, it pays to make a regular habit of eating soups, either as mid-day snacks or as a starter course to a main meal. These can be bought ready made, or prepared at home from leftovers and locally sourced ingredients. (Home-made soups can usually be safely stored in the freezer for up to two months.) By doing this you'll not only lose weight, but also improve your health, save money, and play your part in safeguarding the environment. This was shown by a study of the dustbins of over two thousand volunteers, which revealed that the annual total of jettisoned foodstuffs in Britain has now reached a staggering £10 billion a year. This is not only a waste of valuable food, but also an extravagant misuse of transport facilities, since the merchandise has to be carried to the supermarkets, then to our homes, and from there to the landfill sites and incinerators where it decomposes and releases methane, a highly potent greenhouse gas. If only Britons would turn those edible scraps into soup, they'd reduce the country's emissions of carbon dioxide by an estimated eighteen million tons a year.

Just over twenty years ago researchers at Johns Hopkins University, Baltimore, provided lunch for twelve men for two weeks. On different days the men received one of three hors d'oeuvre dishes before their main course: either tomato soup, cheese and biscuits, or fresh fruit. Each of these appetizers contained exactly the same number of calories, but the follow-up analysis showed that the tomato soup beat the other two starters in reducing the number of calories consumed during the main course. The difference was appreciable, and probably arose because the soup had extra bulk, and so triggered a feeling of satiety by occupying a greater volume of gastric space.

STEP 18

Develop the habit of eating soup, either as a starter before your main meal, or as a pick-me-up snack during the day.

STEP 19

Let There Be Light

The battle against obesity must be waged on many fronts. Scientists of all disciplines must come out of their ivory towers and unite to tackle this growing plague. One area of expertise which has so far been sadly ignored is that of epidemiology. This speciality, which investigates the impact of disease in its environmental setting, is one of the cornerstones of evidence-based public health research. The discipline was born at the start of the nineteenth century, when Dr John Snow investigated an outbreak of cholera in the Soho district of London, and found that the sufferers had all been drinking water from one particular well. He didn't know that cholera was a water-borne bacterial disease, but nevertheless played his hunch and found that the outbreak could be checked by removing the handle from the offending pump. Is there a chance that the science which Dr Snow founded two centuries ago could help us tackle the obesity plague, which is now killing far more people worldwide than all those who once died from infectious diseases, like cholera, smallpox, malaria and typhoid fever?

Obesity rates are rising exponentially throughout the world. In Britain there has been a four-fold increase in the number of overweight adults over the past twenty-five years. Across the waters, the Canadian authorities have reported a surge of roughly five hundred per cent in the incidence of obesity among young boys and girls. But this explosive growth hasn't been evenly spread. Epidemiological studies reveal that obesity is far more common in urban areas than it is in the countryside. This variance is particularly marked in the emerging countries. In China, for instance, the incidence of obesity is four times higher in the cities than it is the vast majority of rural areas. Why should this be? Could country dwellers benefit from spending more time out of doors, sitting down less, enjoying higher levels of physical activity, and being more exposed to the stimulus of fresh air, sunshine and cooling draughts of air?

There seems little doubt that we're at our happiest, and healthiest, when we're out of doors. This was revealed when two British researchers enlisted the help of over six hundred volunteers and asked them to complete an online questionnaire about their mood changes during the previous day. The results showed that the subjects got little pleasure from 'work' and 'shopping'. Most of their enjoyment came from eighteen key activities. These included 'time with children' and 'sex', which both came in the middle of the hedonic ratings, well below 'outdoor activities' which proved to be the No 1 way of achieving a feeling of contentment and well-being. We weren't designed to live indoors, and spend our daylight hours enclosed in man-made boxes. This modus vivendi is far removed from that of our forebears, who lived, worked and played out-of-doors. We've now become prisoners, trapped inside our man-made concrete jungles. Since the start of the Industrial Revolution we've evolved into a strange new species, which might well be dubbed *Homo encapsularis*. This revolutionary lifestyle change has had a subtle, but profound, effect on our outlook, mood and body chemistry. Many people with a tendency to depression find that their moods lift whenever they engage in some form of outdoor activity. This was confirmed recently when a number of British celebrities, who were known to be victims of clinical depression, were asked if they had any pet remedies for escaping the blues. The response of one TV presenter was similar in essence to that of the entire group. 'The first thing I try and do is to get outside. It doesn't matter what weather or time of year it is, it is essential to go out of doors.'

Scientific research strongly suggests that the artificiality of our encapsulated lifestyle is endangering our health, and may well be a hitherto unrecognized factor in our burgeoning rates of obesity. When we're indoors we're kept artificially warm. The moment we step outside we're exposed to cooling breezes which can increase the metabolism of lean subjects by twelve to sixteen per cent. Unfortunately, this is less of a stimulus for the Billie and Bessie Bunters of this world, who are swathed in a duffel coat of fat which provides three times as much insulation against heat loss as lean muscle tissue. A switch from outdoor to indoor living also entails an almost inevitable drop in activity levels. Winston Churchill was always urging his wife to conserve her energy. 'Never stand up when you can sit down, never sit down when you can lie down,' was his regular admonition. Anyone who wants to maintain a healthy weight should do the very opposite, for excess sitting is a health hazard in its own right. When Australian researchers compared the lifestyles and medical records of nearly nine thousand people over a period of six years, they discovered that for each hour per day their subjects spent watching television, their risk of dying from cardiovascular disease rose by eighteen per cent, and their chance of dying from cancer by nine per cent. We become obese if we lead excessively sedentary lives, and use energy only to shift our bodies from car seat to office chair, and then in the evening from car seat to easy chair in front of the TV set.

The other reason for spending more time out of doors is to get an optimum dose of sunshine. People who spend too much time in gloomy rooms show a decline in energy levels, sexual vitality and mental well-being. This cluster of symptoms is now known as Seasonal Affective Disorder, but was once called Lapp Sickness since it afflicts one in every ten people living in northern latitudes. It's a syndrome linked with symptoms of lethargy, a tendency to overeat, and a craving for easily digested carbohydrates. Anyone who follows this pathway will imbibe too many calories and burn up too little energy, which is a sure recipe for putting on weight. We need the regular diurnal variations in light intensity, and the sharp contrast between night and day, to maintain the proper functioning of our hormonal system.

This is best achieved by spending as much time as possible out of doors. At most times of the year in England it's reckoned that a person who spends sixteen hours a day in a typically lit room gets as much light as they would in just one hour outdoors. Even on cloudy days, sunlight is a metabolic stimulus which we all urgently need.

STEP 19
Spend as much time as you can out of doors.

STEP 20

Grow it, Cook it, Eat it

How times have changed! Our forebears spent a large part of their lives foraging for food. Now, in a half hour's rampage through a supermarket, we can get enough food to feed a family of four for an entire week. This change in our way of life is one of the major causes of our current obesity crisis. 'Man is the only animal that consumes without producing,' was George Orwell's take on the situation. 'He does not give milk, he does not lay eggs, he is too weak to pull the plough, he can't run fast enough to catch rabbits.' That is true. Nowadays few of us fish or hunt game. We don't keep pigs and chickens in our backyards, or scavenge the hedgerows for edible fruits, nuts and berries. This has stripped our lives of some of its primordial excitement and challenge. Now that our hunter-gathering is confined to the local supermarket, our fitness levels have dropped, and our body weights have risen. From a medical, and environmental, point of view the Western world would be a far healthier place if we reverted to growing some of our own fruit and vegetables.

This happened from sheer necessity at the start of World War Two, when Britain was importing fifty-five million tons of food a year, much of which came from North and South America. When hostilities began, the Germans launched a U-boat campaign which decimated this supply. The UK government responded by inaugurating a highly successful 'Dig for Victory' crusade, with a campaign song which I well remember: 'Dig! Dig! Dig! And your muscles will grow big.' By the war's end, Britain was producing more than a million tons of vegetables a year, and the nation's health was flourishing as never before. Anyone who wants to lose weight should adopt a similar policy. By growing organic food on our own doorsteps, we'll have access to wholesome fare which is super fresh, free of pesticides and hasn't added to the pollution of the environment by being transported thousands of miles by road and air. (Today, one-fifth of the petrol consumed in America goes on producing and transporting the nation's food.)

One of the first things that Michelle Obama did on entering the White House was to create an organic garden. This she did to promote the cause of healthy eating. If you lack the space to follow her example, rent an allotment. In Britain, at the start of the twentieth century, there was a mass migration from the countryside to the rapidly developing industrial cities. As a consequence farm labourers boosted their earnings, but lost contact with their pastoral roots and close-knit rural communities. This alienation drove some to drink and others to crime. In an attempt to allay these social ills the British government passed an Allotment Act (1908) which made it a duty for all local authorities to provide garden plots for the 'labouring poor'. This edict was largely ignored until the start of the First World War, when the Board of Agriculture was given wide powers to requisition land. Within three years over half a million allotment plots were created in parks, golf courses, tennis courts, abandoned gardens, rubbish tips and railway embankments. Now, once again, we're being urged to grow our own vegetables, not to supplement the country's food supply, but because of the 'therapeutic potential' of gardening as a means of reducing the toll of obesity and coronary disease. This programme has the backing of medical research, which shows that as little as one hour's gardening a week is sufficient to provide substantial protection against sudden cardiac death. If you're not fit enough to dig, maintain a compost heap. This will at least get you out in the open air and make you aware of the endless cycle of life and death. Source your food with care from local farmers' markets. Maintain a well-kempt lawn. A recent NASA study revealed that grass lawns cover forty thousand square miles of America, which makes it the largest of all the country's irrigated 'crops'. Anyone maintaining one of these green handkerchiefs will enjoy an excellent source of regular exercise, for it's reckoned that the average gardener covers a distance of over 220 miles during his or her lifetime mowing their lawn.

With continuing growth in the global population, the UN believes that the world must produce seventy per cent more food by 2050 to prevent major shortages. Some of this shortfall could be made good if individuals were prepared to work their private allotments and gardens, and far more will be generated if urbanites can be persuaded to band together to create city farms and community gardens. (Currently there are over five thousand of these co-operative farmsteads in America, and about a thousand in Britain.) The reward is that anyone who takes up gardening will boost their health and forge a powerful link between food production, healthy eating and sustainable development. This existential bond is particularly important for children, some of whom when quizzed were found to believe that carrots grew above ground, with their tips pointing upwards. 'Food, for many children,' said teachers at one English primary school, 'is something that comes in a packet and is bought from the supermarket.' To raise their awareness of the connection between the natural environment and the food they ate, the teachers started a school gardening club. This was so successful that it led to a countrywide 'Grow it, Cook it, Eat it' initiative, designed to make children more knowledgeable about the foods they eat. As part of this programme one school grew a crop of wheat, which the children ground into flour and then baked into bread. A similar programme was launched in Thailand, when children as young as four and five were encouraged to plant and grow vegetable seeds, take part in fruit and vegetable tasting parties, cook vegetable soups, and watch cartoons of Popeye growing strong through eating lashings of spinach. As a result they doubled their vegetable intake.

Similar benefits are gained by adults. This was shown when two Texas universities combined to carry out a study of almost three hundred men and women over the age of fifty. This showed that gardening improved their mental faculties, increased their 'life satisfaction', heightened their 'zest for life' and made them less likely to 'feel old'. The more we develop a green lifestyle, and become discriminating producers of food, rather than heedless purchasers of off-the-shelf packaged foodstuffs, the healthier and slimmer we'll become.

STEP 20
Rediscover your links with Mother Earth, by playing a more active role in the growing and sourcing of your food.

STEP 21

Don't Fall Foul of
the 'Night Eating Syndrome'

Each of the first twenty steps of the EssVee programme has been explained in splendid isolation, whereas in reality they're very closely interlinked. This is how they get their effectiveness and power, for like a Gobelin tapestry, they're all part of one interwoven fabric. Some weeks ago, when stressing the importance of starting the day with a substantial breakfast, we quoted the old South American maxim: 'Eat breakfast like a king, lunch like a princess and dinner like a pauper.' More recently, when extolling the benefits of the Nibbler's diet, we explained why it's unwise to limit one's intake of nourishment to one or two large meals. This week we examine these principles in greater depth.

One novel way of losing weight is to see what people do when they want to boost their bulk by artificial means, and then do the very opposite. For instance, there's much to be learnt by observing the technique employed by the grotesquely obese Japanese Sumo wrestlers. They go without breakfast, then eat an enormous lunch and immediately afterwards retire to bed so that the calories they've gorged have the maximum chance of being turned to fat. That's a practice to avoid. We've suggested previously that it's wise to start the day by eating a hearty breakfast, and to keep hunger pangs at bay by taking several light snacks throughout the day. Building on that platform, this week's assignment is to avoid eating a heavy meal last thing at night. This is a mistake that many people make, some getting eighty per cent of their daily calorie intake at night. Their days are filled with work, which means that they have little time to eat during the day. By the time they come home in the evening they're ravenous, so they're driven to tuck into a hefty meal. As a result their blood sugar level soars. This stimulates the release of extra insulin which takes the glucose out of the circulation and conveys it to the body's fat stores. That can easily lead to a spell of rebound hypoglycaemia, which provokes them to snack eat while they're reading a book or watching TV. After that they go to bed, unconsciously copying the obesogenic tactics of the Sumo wrestlers.

This failing was first made the subject of serious study in the 1950s, when Dr Albert 'Mickey' Stunkard, a trainee psychiatrist at the New York Medical Center, encountered a girl who had an unusual pattern of eating. She overate enormously, but was never hungry in the morning, and ate relatively little throughout the day. But the moment night fell she felt an overwhelming need to eat. This she did voraciously, a compulsion so strong that it kept her awake. As she tossed and turned, she comforted herself by further munching. Unable to make sense of her obsessive behaviour, he sought the help of his colleagues at a routine, case-sharing conference. One of the group, who was herself decidedly obese, grew clearly upset as he gave details of the girl's bizarre behaviour. Finally, she admitted that she herself was a victim of the same compulsion. This led Mickey Stunkard to make a detailed study of what he eventually came to call the 'Night Eating Syndrome'. At the start of his enquiry, he investigated twenty-five obese patients, who'd been referred for psychiatric treatment because they'd failed to lose weight by standard dietary treatment. On close questioning, he found that every one of them skipped breakfast, and all consumed at least a quarter of their daily calories *after* their evening meal. He decided that this unhealthy aberration was a response to stress, which disturbed their sleep and provoked the urge to comfort eat the moment the lights went down and they were left alone with their thoughts in the wee, small hours of the night. He was one of the pioneers of lifestyle weight reduction, telling his peers in a paper published in 1957 in the *American Journal of Surgery*: 'Many physicians and their patients who had formerly looked upon weight reduction as a cosmetic conceit have now come to consider it as a therapeutic imperative.'

Dr Stunkard had to overcome one fallacious folk belief before his concepts were finally accepted. This was the old wives' tale that people should eat a substantial meal before they retired to bed for fear of suffering 'night starvation'. This idea was probably a hangover from the days when many people were chronically undernourished, a state which does indeed cause restless sleep. This is why insomnia is a common complaint of anorexic patients, who invariably sleep more soundly when they resume a normal pattern of eating. It's unwise to be ravenously hungry when you go to bed, and equally foolish to take a heavy meal. A bedtime mug of malted milk may help you sleep, but anything more substantial is likely to have the opposite effect, and add to your weight problems. Ideally the last activity at night should be, not eating, but gentle exercise. Whenever you can, bring your day to a close by taking a leisurely walk around the block. This will relax your muscles and boost your metabolic rate, so that you'll continue to burn up calories even after you fall asleep. All of which is in line with the old proverb: 'After lunch sit a while, after supper walk a mile.'

STEP 21
Eat a light evening meal, followed if possible by a little gentle exercise, then you won't fall victim to the Night Eating Syndrome.

STEP 22

Don't Allow Yourself to Become a Sugar Junkie

The major premise of this book is that the world's obesity plague is the product of a dramatic change in our habits and way of life. A clear example of this is our increased consumption of refined sugar, a craving which has rocketed sky-high in the last two hundred years. People throughout the developed world have become sugar junkies. This addiction is easily explained, for sugar activates the brain's pleasure centres in exactly the same way as psychedelic drugs. It also helps us cope with stress. This was shown when scientists from the University of New South Wales, Australia, subjected young rats to stress by separating them from their mothers. Subsequently it was found that those who were placated with sweets, biscuits and cakes made a speedier recovery from their anxiety state than those who continued to eat their normal, unexciting rodent fare. Sugar has the same soothing effect on other animals, especially when they're young.

Nowadays, from the moment human infants are born we train them to develop a sweet tooth habit. As babies, we pacify them with dummies soaked in honey. When they grow up to be toddlers, we give them sweeties to stop them crying. Then, as youngsters, we reward them for joining us on boring supermarket shopping excursions by allowing them to make impulse buys from the tempting array of candy at the checkout counter. We teach them that if they're good, mummy will give them a sweetie. This behavioural conditioning is now deeply engrained in our psyches. It's a ploy that's been used since the beginning of recorded time; a reward that Jewish fathers traditionally gave their sons when

83

they were diligent in their Torah studies. This is recorded in an Old Testament instruction, which says that young boys studying hard for their bar mitzvah should be rewarded by having their palates rubbed with chewed dates.

Both our nature, and our nurture, encourage us to become sugar addicts. This was noted by William Duffy, the prize-winning American writer who became a powerful leader of the anti-sucrose movement. This came about after a chance encounter with the legendary film star Gloria Swanson. Sitting beside her at the end of a New York meeting, he followed his usual practice of sweetening his coffee with a generous helping of sugar. Much to his surprise, the actress leaned across and whispered in his ear: 'That stuff is poison. I won't have it in my house, let alone my body.' Swanson was sixteen years his senior but still in marvellous condition, whereas he at the time was decidedly plump, a short but hefty sixteen stone. After chatting to her for some while he decided to take her advice and quit eating sugar. Some years later they met again, when he was infinitely fitter and six stone lighter. Their friendship blossomed, and he became her sixth and final husband. This transforming experience motivated him to write what became a best-selling book *Sugar Blues* (1975), in which he argued that sugar, like morphine and heroin, is an addictive, self-destructive drug. The book got its title because he noted that sugar addicts often experience brief bouts of despondency, fatigue and irritability after eating heavily sweetened foods. These symptoms arise when an intake of sucrose triggers a release of insulin followed by a sudden spell of rebound hypogly-caemia, which leaves the body temporarily deplete of get-up-and-go.

Professor John Yudkin, one of the founding fathers of nutritional medicine, was another potent anti-sugar campaigner. As Director of International Health and Medical Education at University College Hospital, London, he and his team of researchers carried out a series of experiments which showed the health risks of eating too much concentrated sugar. This practice leads to a sudden rise in insulin levels, which takes the excess glucose out of the circulation and converts it into fats, which are immediately deposited in the body's fat stores. It also inhibits the release of growth hormones, which in turn depress the immune system. Other tests carried out by his team revealed that sugar-rich diets predispose to dermatitis, liver disease and a reduction in the life expectancy of laboratory animals. On the basis of these findings, Yudkin wrote an influential, chart-topping book *Pure, White and Deadly* (1972). In this he asserted that there was no physical requirement whatsoever for us to eat refined sugar. In fact, he pronounced: 'If only a small fraction of what is already known about the effects of sugar were to be revealed in relation to any other material used as a food additive, that material would promptly be banned.' Despite these powerful warnings, the people of the developed nations continue to fill their stomachs with artificially sweetened foodstuffs. This is making them fat, and predisposing them to a wide range of chronic ailments ranging from dental decay to diabetes, coronary disease, cancer and premature death. The average person who shuns all forms of sugar-sweetened foods can expect to lose about a pound of unwanted fat a week, and save enough money in the course of a year to treat themselves to a weekend holiday treat.

STEP 22
Reduce your intake of sugar and artificially sweetened foods to an absolute minimum.

STEP 23

Fizzy Drinks and Fuzzy Figures

We live today in a global village. We're part of multi-ethnic community which circles the world, but is nevertheless heavily influenced by American mores and culture. Every continent imports US movies and TV shows. Computer operating systems, generated by Microsoft and other Silicon Valley companies, are used throughout the globe. People, whatever their native tongues, gain information from Wikipedia, and search engines like Google and Yahoo. They communicate with their friends through social websites like Facebook and Twitter, all of which originated in the USA. What America does today, the rest of the world is likely do tomorrow. This cultural dominance has its downside, for the nation which has spread its breathtaking, man-on-the-moon technology has also transmitted its lifestyle diseases. It's given the world Superman and Mickey Mouse, but it's also exported its sugar-laden fizzy drinks which have spread the obesity plague as surely as mosquitoes spread malaria. Under its influence the world has been Coca-colanized.

It all began so very innocently. In the eighteenth century wealthy Europeans travelled to the elegant spa towns of Bath, Carlsbad and Baden-Baden to drink the sparkling spa waters, which were widely believed to have healing properties. To make these medicinal waters available to the less affluent, Joseph Priestley, the English dissident priest and part-time scientist, invented a way of making artificial carbonated drinks. This technology was eventually exported to America, where it was widely adopted by small town pharmacies which attracted customers by providing soda fountains. These became a popular part of the US social scene in the nineteenth century, when people would gather in the local pharmacy for a glass of soda pop, just as they call in today to a Starbuck's café to meet their friends over a leisurely cup of cappuccino. In 1893 one of these chemists, by the name of Caleb Bradham, started to sell a special health drink in his pharmacy which contained the enzyme pepsin to aid digestion, and kola nuts to provide an energy boost. The drink was an immediate success. Originally known as 'Brad's drink', it was later given the name of its ingredients – Pepsi-Cola. It was then the troubles started, for the fizzy drink was soon laden with sugar to enhance its appeal and boost its sales. This brought about a rapid transformation, turning a local health drink into an international health hazard. Today there are two rival products – Pepsi-Cola and Coca-Cola – which are both sweetened with high-fructose corn syrup. This turns them into unwholesome, highly addictive drinks, which the US Center for Science in the Public Interest has aptly described as 'Liquid Candy'. In a report published in 1998, the Center provided evidence which showed that the consumption of these sugar-sweetened soft drinks predisposes to obesity, type 2 diabetes, dental decay and poor overall nutrition. It may or may not be a coincidence, but over the last two decades of the twentieth century Americans doubled their consumption of these sugar-laden drinks, a trend which was paralleled by a doubling of the nation's obesity rates. Now, these drinks provide a quarter of the daily calorie intake of the average young American. Delete them from their menu, and the problem of childhood obesity would be solved.

Few realize just how addictive sugar drinks can be. This was demonstrated in 2001, when two American neuroscientists gave laboratory rats the chance of sipping sugar syrup similar in concentration to that contained in a typical cola drink. This they were offered alongside their normal food supply. After a month on the cola candy, the rats developed behaviour and brain changes which were identical to those shown by their litter mates who were addicted to morphine. They binged compulsively on the syrup and showed signs of withdrawal when it was no longer available. The overuse of these alluring, sugar-saturated drinks is now a major cause of obesity, for studies show that people who drink an extra two fluid ounces of these drinks each day will increase their weight by about three pounds a year. This is causing major problems in many Third World countries, where the drinks are popular because they offer a cheap source of calories. Mexico is a poor country, yet it now has the third highest consumption of Coke and Pepsi-Cola in the world. Not surprisingly, well over two-thirds of its adult population is now overweight. As a result, the Mexican government is considering putting a tax on all sweetened soft drinks and imposing a complete ban on their TV advertising.

There is no doubt that these heavily marketed drinks pose a major health risk. An eight-year investigation of fifty thousand female nurses revealed that women who increased their consumption of soft drinks gained eight kilograms during the course of the study. The more they drank the greater their gain. Even worse is the effect this liquid candy is having on children, who are reckoned to be drinking thirty times more colas than they did in 1950. This is making them obese and will also increase their risk of developing cancer in later life, according to a study of over ten thousand students at Bristol University who were measured and weighed at the university's health centre between 1948 and 1968. The results showed that for every eleven pounds the students were overweight, the risk of developing cancer rose by eighty per cent in women and thirty-six per cent in men. A yet more surprising finding is that women who take too many cola drinks may increase their risk of developing gout, a disease which was previously more commonly associated with men. This warning was raised by a study of nearly seventy-five thousand women, which revealed that those who drank more than two sweetened sodas a day were two to four times more likely to develop gout that those who rarely touched the stuff.

If you haven't yet developed a taste for fizzy drinks, be grateful. You've won brownie points and this week will have no habit change to make. This will give you time to make sure that your children and grandchildren don't become addicted to liquid candy drinks. Studies show that about seventy per cent of adolescents are regular consumers of fizzy drinks, which means they have a calorie intake which is on average ten per cent higher than those who don't. Get them to cut down, and you'll have played your part in protecting the health of the coming generation. If they want to slake their thirst, encourage them to eat an apple, for they'd have to eat four large apples to get the calories in a small glass of pop.

STEP 23
Stop drinking colas and other fizzy drinks laden with sugar.

STEP 24

Waterways to Weight Control

Man evolved from the sea, and despite aeons of evolutionary development we still retain that aquatic link. Our bodies have a solid feel, yet in fact they remain roughly two-thirds water. No single human function – from creating new cells to controlling our internal body temperature – can take place without this life-giving fluid. Water is our most vital nutrient, and yet it's rarely ever considered in relation to physical fitness and weight control. To satisfy our metabolic requirements we need to consume about four pints of water a day. If we drink less and become dehydrated our efficiency shows a dramatic decline. Sports physiologists have found that a five per cent loss of body fluid is sufficient to produce a fifteen per cent decline in all-round athletic performance. One simple way of satisfying this vital nutritional need is to adopt the habit of taking a leisurely glass of water before every meal. This has the added advantage of creating a feeling of satiety, which makes us less likely to eat to excess during the meal which follows. Our ancestors lived on diets rich in fruit and vegetables which have a high fluid content. This satisfied their fluid needs, and at the same slaked their hunger by filling their bellies with fibrous foods low in calorie content. We, on the other hand, exist on concentrated foodstuffs which are stuffed with calories, sugars and fats, but contain relatively little fluid.

Recent research suggests that this dietary change could be fooling our bodies into eating far more than they really need. Dr George Blackburn, director of the Center for the Study of Nutritional Medicine at Harvard Medical School, is one of the increasing band of nutritionists who believe that what the brain today interprets as hunger may sometimes actually be thirst. This would not be surprising, since the brain centres responsible for the regulation of hunger and thirst are situated close together in the brain stem. If this theory is true, then it would seem wise to satisfy the body's demand for water before we sate its need for food. If nothing else, this would speed the filling of our stomachs and reduce our tendency to bolt our food.

In practice, we're hopeless at gauging our calorie intake. Researchers proved this when they asked hungry volunteers to drink an entire meal supplied as a chocolate liquid. This was fed to them through a straw from an opaque container, so they had no idea what exactly they were drinking. The liquid always felt and tasted the same, even though the experiment was planned so that its calorie content varied ten-fold. Despite this wide variation in the energy content of the drinks, the subjects always drank the same amount. Clearly, it was the volume of liquid that made them feel satiated and not its calorie content. This means that a glass of water is likely to be just as filling as a swig of Red Bull or Coca-Cola. In the 1930s many health gurus suggested that it was unwise to drink before a meal, because it diluted the gastric juices and so impaired the process of digestion. This is now known to be untrue. In fact recent physiological studies have shown that a pre-dinner drink of water acts as a mild stimulus to the flow of gastric juices.

Many people put on weight during the winter months, and it's possible that this may also be due in part to an inadequate intake of liquid. If there's any validity in Dr Blackburn's hypothesis, we may overeat in the winter to satisfy a thirst created by our overheated indoor environments. This can cause an unhygienic drop in the humidity levels in our homes and offices. Even in the most arid deserts, the relative humidity rarely drops below twenty to thirty per cent. During the winter in overheated, draught-proofed rooms it's not uncommon for it to fall as low as three to five per cent. In these parched conditions furniture warps, indoor plants wilt, pianos go out of tune and the skin and mucous membranes of our eyes, nose and throat grow dry.

We become dehydrated, and if we don't take steps to slake our thirst we may well be fooled into overeating. This is particularly important for the over-fifties, for thirst perception diminishes with age and continues to decline the older we get.

At one time, when mothers were bottle-feeding their babies they were advised to give them water first to quench their thirst, then milk to satisfy their hunger. There is now scientific evidence to back the adoption of this practice. This is based on research carried out by Brenda Davy, a nutritional scientist at Virginia Tech, Blacksburg, Virginia, who put a group of would-be slimmers on an identical low-calorie diet. Half the group was asked to drink two small glasses of water before their meals, the others ate their food without any prior attempt to quench their thirst. The results showed that at the end of the twelve-week period the water drinkers had lost an average of seven kilograms compared with the control group which had lost two kilograms less. Of even greater significance, for the purposes of our EssVee programme, when the volunteers were followed up at a later stage, it was found that those who'd maintained the water-drinking habit were significantly better at maintaining their weight loss.

If you find water a trifle bland, try the experiment of drinking green tea before the occasional meal whenever time permits. Trials carried out at the University of Geneva, Switzerland, reveal that green tea contains antioxidant chemicals known as catechin polyphenols. These raise the metabolic rate and so increase the rate at which surplus calories are consumed. In a randomized trial of ten healthy young men, those who unknowingly took green tea capsules showed a four per cent increase in metabolic rate and overall energy consumption.

STEP 24
Satisfy your thirst, and curb your appetite, by taking a leisurely glass of water before your meals.

STEP 25

Tripping the Light Fantastic

Fifty years ago I met the eminent English-born anthropologist Francis Huxley. He'd just returned from the Amazon basin, where he'd been living in intimate contact with some of the indigenous tribes who'd previously had no contact whatsoever with the outside world. Out of curiosity I asked him: 'What are the main differences you found in the lifestyles of these native people and those living in the developed countries?' After a moment's reflection he replied: 'There are two main distinctions. First they touch each more than we do; and secondly they make far more use of dancing to express their feelings and celebrate the major events in their tribal life.'

Dancing is a universal language spoken across the globe. Every culture has its own particular ethnic dance, when neighbours join together to socialize and make merry. Even in a country as small as Britain the tradition varies from region to region. The Scots take part in energetic Highland reels, the Irish favour clog dancing, while the English – if they're in party mood – may join in a Conga or dance to the Cockney song of 'Knees up Mother Brown'. Observant tourists, when they travel round the world, will encounter every conceivable form of choreography, from belly dancing to lindy hops, salsas, tangos and cha cha chas. We may not understand what foreigners are saying when they speak, but we immediately recognize the mood they're in when they dance.

Dancing generates joy and it also burns up calories. Michelle Obama, America's First Lady, is a great fan of dancing as a means of keeping fit, and gave a public demonstration of its value when she was pictured on the White

House lawns dancing freely to a Beyoncé song with a party of eighty very happy children. Professional dancers find it almost impossible to put on weight. One British performer drank a glass of sugar syrup every night to get a part as a dancing fatty-puff in the West End musical *Me and My Girl*. As the show went on he found it more and more difficult to maintain his bulk. When the show closed he found he'd been typecast, and was called upon to build himself up for a similar role in *Crazy for You*. After appearing in nine shows a week for six months he found he'd lost a stone in weight. Once again he had to force feed himself like a Strasbourg goose to satisfy the casting director's requirements. 'It's the hours of tap dancing that has done it,' he ruefully explained.

Dancing is a conditioning exercise suitable for people of all ages and levels of physical fitness. Some years ago a ten-day 'Festival of the Aged' was held in Bulgaria, when well over a thousand people from eighty upwards joined together to dance the night away and celebrate their geriatric health and fitness. Fifty-six of the participants were over a hundred, yet no serious mishaps were reported. In fact many heart specialists now recommend dancing as a pleasurable way of recovering from cardiac disease. One Mexican specialist told his colleagues, gathered at a World Congress of Cardiology, that he'd offered patients recuperating from coronary attacks and heart-valve surgery the choice of building up their strength by either dancing, or working out on a static bicycle. Those who opted to dance improved their heart health and exercise capacity by a massive twenty-eight per cent. Dancing has an added benefit for the elderly, as was shown when researchers at the Geneva Faculty of Medicine took a group of well over a hundred volunteers, and set them the task of exercising to music for just one hour a week over a period of six months. This improved their balance and more than halved the number of falls they suffered.

The more you find time to dance, the healthier and slimmer you'll become. This has been the experience of the celebrity contestants taking part in the TV show *Strictly Come Dancing*. Pamela Stephenson, the sex therapist who is probably best known as the wife of Billy Connolly, lost two stone and dropped two dress sizes during the course of the competition, which she describes as 'The best fat camp in the universe ... I am the fittest I've ever been in my life.' The actress Patsy Kensit admits that she put on masses of weight after the end of her fourth marriage. By taking part in the show she lost two stone, regained her confidence, and no longer feels the need to comfort eat. 'Dancing changes the way you hold yourself, your posture and actually how you feel about yourself,' she told reporters. 'You get something from it that you wouldn't get if you just went to the gym.' Even Ann Widdecombe, the chubby 62-year-old ex-politician, dropped two dress sizes during the first few weeks of the show. She'd struggled with a weight problem throughout her life, and by dancing achieved a result that she'd failed to gain from all the standard crash dieting programmes, including Weight Watchers and the Atkins Diet. The same applies to the stars who took part in *Dancing with the Stars*, the American version of the show. Kelly Osborne, who is described as a British singer and fashion designer, lost fourteen pounds in the first six weeks of training. The same applied to the thirty-year-old Mya, the US hip hop singer/songwriter, who lost eleven pounds in four weeks and said that, although she always kept fit through running, she now found that: 'My body has gotten more toned. I'm seeing a lot more definition.' Commenting on these changes, Sarah Dussault, a leading US fitness trainer said: 'Dancing is arguably one of the most efficient methods of physical activity for weight loss.' Anyone who goes to a dance class, and performs a strenuous dance like a hip hop, can expect to lose six hundred calories in a single hour.

Dancing should once more become part of our culture and private daily routines. Maybe we should adopt the custom of Lila and DeWitt Wallace, the founders of the *Reader's Digest*, who always danced together before they retired to bed. Whenever you've got a moment to spare freak out, play some music and express your feelings through bodily movement. Socrates was in the habit of dancing on his own. Likewise many Chinese, who had a tradition of making tiny dance steps to follow the delicate patterning of their carpets. We too should find time to turn on the music and dance. Then we'll find the joy and tranquillity that the philosopher Schopenhauer said all animals experience when they consider neither past nor future but live only in the immediate present.

STEP 25
Every day, try to find time to dance.

STEP 26

Don't be a Slavish Follower of Fashion

Keeping slim is largely a matter of habit. That's the leitmotif of this book, as by now you've probably gathered. Life is unpredictable and sometimes positively hazardous. To make it safer for beginners, children are trained to abide by a number of simple, safety-first precautions. Some of these are sound, but others are unscientific and well past their sell-by date. One of these dangerous shibboleths is the belief that we should devour every scrap of food that's placed before us. That in my youth was a widely held working-class tradition. Children of labourers were taught to clean their plates completely 'or you'll know want', whereas upper-class youngsters were trained to leave something on the plate for 'Mr Manners', which demonstrated that they were neither greedy, nor starving. Among primitive people, the demand to eat every scrap of food was equally firmly enforced. It was instigated by the shamans, who were the tribal healers and priests. They wanted their kinsfolk to overeat to build up their fat stores in preparation for future spells of famine. So they spread the myth that any particles of food they left would be devoured by hobgoblins and evil spirits, who as a result would grow stronger and so more capable of causing them harm. This pagan belief still lingers on in the Christian rite of Holy Communion, when priests are trained to consume every unused hallowed wafer lest they're eaten by Satan and serve to increase his wicked, supernatural powers. Some devout Catholics still believe that wasting food is sinful, a view supported by a Catholic priest who tells on his blog how he was brought up in poverty and trained by his mother to 'clean his plate'. Failure to do so he still regards as a venial sin, which can only be expunged by the rites of confession and absolution. But isn't gluttony a far greater offence?

The idea of licking the platter clean gained strength and credibility in the West during the two world wars, when food was in short supply. Herbert Hoover, head of the US Food Administration, started the ball rolling at the start of World War I when he launched a 'Clean Plate' campaign. This encouraged children to make a sincere and public pledge: 'At table I'll not leave a scrap of food upon my plate.' This idea was revived in the 1939–45 war, when President Harry Truman launched a 'Clean Plates Club', which urged children to clear their plates to help the starving in Europe. While this was being done in America, the British people were being exhorted to adopt the same economy. Parents coaxed their children to be good boys and girls by finishing their meals, even when they were already full. If that failed, an appeal was made to their conscience. They were made to feel guilty, by being reminded of the millions of children who were starving in Third World countries. Outright threats were made if these pleas failed: 'If you don't clear that plate tonight you'll have it for breakfast.' These strict admonitions were backed by a publicity campaign, financed by the UK Ministry of Food which issued posters declaring 'A clear plate is a clear conscience'.

We're now in a totally different situation, for we live in a world of surfeit rather than shortage. Yet the old habit remains. We still feel the need to clean our plates, which we're now told we must do to save the planet. But what earthly good does it do if we save the world and in the process shorten our own lives? This is a grave risk today, for an average serving of French fries is now twice the size it was at the end of World War I. Psychological studies reveal that we're now eating, not to satisfy our hunger, but simply to clean our plates. In one trial a band of student volunteers was split into two groups, both of which were served lunch in their college canteen. The only difference was that one of the sets was consistently given a larger helping of food.

Despite this marked variation, they all cleared their platters just as they'd been trained to do as children. What's more, when quizzed afterwards, both groups reported similar feelings of satiation. In another research project, groups of four volunteers were invited to sit down together at a cafeteria table which had already been laid out with four bowls of soup. Unbeknown to the subjects, two of the bowls had been ingeniously doctored so that they could be replenished surreptitiously from a container concealed beneath the table. In this way the participants were fooled into drinking seventy-three per cent more soup than the controls. Nevertheless, when asked how full they felt, they made exactly the same estimate as those who'd drunk the lesser amount. This was a consistent finding whenever the experiment was repeated, whatever the subject's sex, age or body build, which led the researchers to conclude they were merely following the instruction they'd been given as children, to carry on eating until their plates were cleared.

This is a particular hazard when we're eating out, and feel compelled to eat whatever is put before us. Even when we're full, we feel compelled to eat the last scrap of pizza or hamburger bought from fast food cafés. The same applies when we sit down to a three-course restaurant meal. One diner ate his starter dish and entrée and then told the waiter that he hadn't room for anything more. The server tried to tempt him to eat a light dessert, suggesting maybe a caramel custard or fresh fruit salad. 'No,' the man insisted, 'I couldn't manage another mouthful.' Seconds later he quickly changed his mind, when he was reminded that the dessert was included in the price of the meal. 'In that case I'll have the sticky toffee pudding – with ice cream.' Many professional chefs offer their clients quantity rather than quality and can't tolerate waste. The owner of a Japanese restaurant in Australia, in a declared attempt to save the planet, even goes so far as to offer her customers a thirty per cent discount if they polish off everything on their plate. To back up this inducement, her waiters are encouraged to tell customers who don't clean their plate to eat elsewhere next time. Misguided attempts like this are fuelling the obesity crisis. Melanie Polk, Director of Nutritional Education at the American Institute of Cancer Research, reports that surveys show that nearly seven out of every ten Americans are members of the 'Clean Plate Club', and so at risk of becoming obese. One of her tips, which you might follow with benefit, is: 'At table service restaurants, ask the server to put half of your entrée in a doggie bag before bringing it to your table.' This strategy will be good for your purse as well as your paunch, for it provides two full meals for the price of one.

STEP 26

Never feel obliged to clear your plate, but stop eating the moment your appestat tells you you've had enough.

STEP 27

Stripping the Power of the Demon Temptation

'Every moment of every day we're surrounded by temptation,' as we observed in Step 10. This makes obesity a far greater problem for people who are easily lured, than it is for those with a high degree of self control. This was the failing of Oscar Wilde, who grew so 'enormously fat' that he had to walk with the aid of an enormous walking stick. His weakness, as he admitted in one of his most famous bon mots, was: 'I can resist everything but temptation.' Today, the enticement to overeat is greater than it has ever been before. Every hour of every day we're exposed to media advertisements tempting us to eat more than we need, or can comfortably afford. The big food stores, knowing that we like to fill our supermarket trolleys to the full, to demonstrate our foresight and affluence, are now boosting their sales by providing larger shopping trolleys. To encourage us to buy more than we really need, they're making far more use of special promotions, bargain offers and two-for-one sales. Somehow we must generate the will-power to resist these lures. This tests our resolve and puts us at risk. If we succeed, we feel good. If we fail, we feel miserable.

Scientists are doing their very best to understand the root causes of our obesity plague. The very least we can do is keep an eye on their investigations, and learn the practical lessons that stem from their research. These include fascinating discoveries in the field of human decision making. Through these studies we've derived a far better understanding of the interrelationship between the workings of our conscious and subconscious minds. It's been found, for instance, that our rational brain, which allows us to make carefully considered decisions, operates only five per cent of the time and has a relatively limited operational capacity, being able to process only forty to sixty bits of information per second. This makes it far less influential than our subconscious brain which operates most of the time and is capable of processing an estimated eleven million bits of information every second. Knowing these figures, it's easy to see the overriding importance of the unconscious mind in determining our food choices. This is why the food industry chooses to speak, not to our reason, but to our passions. Studies have shown that whenever people are shown pictures of food – whether on TV advertisements, roadside hoardings or food packages – they secrete the neurotransmitter dopamine. This triggers a craving to eat, in precisely the same way as our appestats do when we're genuinely hungry. Exactly the same signals are sent out, and the identical control centres of the brain are employed. Overweight people are particularly prone to succumb to these inducements, tests having shown that they're more sensitive to cues in their environment than their slimmer counterparts. The depth analysts have found, for instance, that if background German military music is played in a food store, the sale of German wines will be boosted. In the same way, the sale of French burgundies can be increased by the subliminal broadcasting of Gallic folk tunes played on an accordion.

Another study, carried out by researchers at Cornell University, exposed the role played by 'food visibility'. The team tested forty women and found that they were twice as likely to eat chocolates they could see, as those that were hidden from their view, which proved that mummy was right when she said that our eyes were often bigger than our bellies. The temptation was also reduced when the chocolates were placed six feet from the subjects' work stations rather than within arm's reach. This reduced their nibbling by a full seventy per cent. Given these tendencies, I have every sympathy for the wag who saw a large placard outside a nonconformist church bearing the biblical slogan, 'Lead us not into Temptation', and underneath had scribbled: 'Tell us where it is and we'll find it.' If you're struggling to lose weight, have nothing around you that's easy to eat. If you're fond of nuts, make sure they remain in their shells, for then you'll eat them in far smaller quantities. And keep well away from enticing food smells. Psychologists at the University of Southampton have discovered that fat people have a greater than normal sensitivity to the smell of food, especially towards the end of a meal. This means they should make a conscious habit of leaving the table while they still have room for more, following the example of the Japanese who observe the rule of *hara hachi*, which means 'eat until you're eighty per cent full'. In addition, since we're heavily influenced by our peers, we should ignore the example of Caesar who, in Shakespeare's words said: 'Let me have men about me that are fat.' Instead you should choose to associate, and particularly eat, with people who are slim, for then you're likely to ape their behaviour and eventually acquire a figure which is every bit as svelte as theirs. You must also to learn to say 'No!', for friends will always be offering you something to eat, which is a traditional hospitality gesture throughout the world.

Since it's never too early or late to learn, these are lessons children should be taught as soon as they're able to read, mark and learn. They must be trained to recognize the rewards of deferred gratification. This was shown by the Marshmallow Test, in which four-year-old children were offered a choice which assessed their powers of self control. Either they could eat a marshmallow immediately, or they could carry out a brief errand after which they'd be given *two* marshmallows. Some grabbed the chance of getting the immediate satisfaction, while others managed to hold out for the delayed reward, some only by covering their eyes, singing to themselves or playing games. The children were then retested when they reached high school, when teachers and parents agreed that the children who had originally had the self-discipline to pursue a policy of deferred gratification grew up to be better adjusted teenagers. They were found to be more popular, adventurous and dependable, and showed greater self-confidence, than their greedier primary school classmates, who grew up to be shyer, more easily frustrated and less able to cope with stress This suggests that if we teach our children the Habits of Health, we'll not only help to keep them slim, but also train them to develop into happy, healthy human beings.

STEP 27
Learn the behavioural skills which will help you overcome the temptation to overeat.

STEP 28

The Magic of Mirth

Medical science is growing at an exponential rate. Every year new specialities are being launched. The latest kid on the block is gelotology, which is the study of laughter and the effect it has on the function of the human body. (The term is derived from *geloto*, the Greek word for laughter.) Scientists previously thought this topic too frivolous to warrant their attention. Now, at last, it's recognized that laughter is a powerful medicine, a recipe for longevity and a sure cure for tension and anxiety. Most of all, it helps to oil the wheels of social intercourse. When we laugh, we signal to those around us that all is well. There's no danger on the horizon, so it's safe for everyone in earshot to relax, let their hair down and enjoy themselves in a carefree, uninhibited way. This explains why laughter is so infectious. Laugh and the world laughs with you. By its very nature laughter helps break down the barriers between people, or as the late Victor Borge, the comic concert pianist, put it: 'Laughter is the shortest distance between two people.' You can't be sure that a barking dog won't bite, but you can be pretty confident that a laughing man won't turn and stab you in the back. If we want to spread the brotherhood of man, we'd have far more success if we transmitted peals of laughter round the globe rather than corps of diplomats and politicians. World peace would be more easily achieved by throwing custard pies than by tossing Molotov cocktails.

Laughter also helps us cope during times of stress. In the good times we laugh from pleasure, in the bad times we laugh from sheer necessity. When we're engaged in light-hearted, mirthful activities we relax, which improves our circulation and boosts our blood levels of 'good' cholesterol.

This was shown when a research team at Loma Linda University, California, took a small sample of patients with a high risk of developing heart disease and divided them into two groups. The first was given cholesterol-lowering drugs, while the second was set the therapy of spending half-an-hour a day watching comedy films and TV shows. At the end of a year it was found that the drug takers had increased their 'good' cholesterol levels by just three per cent, whereas the gigglers had boosted theirs by a massive twenty-six per cent.

By raising our mood, laughing also reduces our tendency to comfort eat. In one trial it was found that severely depressed people ate on average twice as many sweets as those who are habitually cheerful. That's because laughter stimulates the production of endorphins in the hypothalamus, the area of the brain which is also involved in appetite regulation. This naturally occurring hormone eases pain and raises mood. Clearly it's better to have a belly laugh than a belly ache, which all too often leads to comfort eating and the development of a belly bulge. This was shown a few years ago, when a study of over six hundred teenage boys and girls revealed that negative moods were linked to increased emotional eating, the boys tending to consume more calories when they were stressed, the girls when they were feeling lonely or low. The tragedy is that at these times comfort eating did little to boost their mood, but rather led to a demoralizing sense of failure and shame.

As well as reducing the tendency to comfort eat, laughter also makes a direct contribution to weight loss. This was shown when researchers at Vanderbilt University, Tennessee, took a group of forty-five young adults and set them the task of watching clips of television shows depicting either comedies or nature films. The results showed a significant increase in energy output when the comedy clips were viewed. According to the team in their concluding report: 'Participants in our study showed a ten to twenty per cent higher energy expenditure during episodes of laughter than during rest.' As a result it was calculated that fifteen minutes' extra chuckling every day could lead to a weight loss of just over four and a half pounds a year. This is probably because it increases our intake of oxygen, boosts our metabolism, makes our chest and diaphragm rise and fall, and gives our abdominal muscles a thorough workout.

Nowadays it's not politically correct to laugh at people with physical disabilities, but previous generations thought it perfectly acceptable to mock people who cared so little for their health that they overindulged, and allowed themselves to become obscenely overweight. Lord Derby was a very obese London nobleman, who'd just finished presiding over a packed meeting in the City's financial centre. The man who had been deputed to show appreciation for his services rose to his feet and declared: 'I have been asked to propose the vote of thanks to Lord Derby for taking the chair, but I really feel I ought to be proposing a vote of thanks to the chair for taking Lord Derby.' This led to peals of laughter from the audience, and the shameful deflation of the honourable stout party. At the other end of the social spectrum, a very large Cockney lady was trying to get through a narrow doorway. An onlooker suggested she tried getting in sideways. 'I ain't got no sideways,' she replied. I think it would help if overweight people learnt to laugh at themselves, acknowledging their problem and making it an object of fun rather than one of denial and guilt. As one psychiatrist observed: 'I've seldom been called upon to help a person who had a sense of the ridiculous, and I've never had to treat anyone who could really laugh at themselves.'

One thing is sure, you can't overeat when you're laughing. So, if you're overweight, try to eat a little less and laugh a whole lot more, for this, in the words of the writer Henry Ward Beecher, is 'God's medicine'.

> **STEP 28**
> Fill your day with laughter and you'll burn up surplus calories and reduce your urge to comfort eat.

STEP 29

The Stress Factor

It's not only hunger that makes us eat, it's also anxiety and fear. Our forebears lived in an environment which was infinitely more dangerous than ours, but the periods of stress they suffered were relatively short-lived. A caveman came face to face with a sabre-toothed tiger, but his time of panic was quickly over. Either he climbed a tree, clubbed the beast to death or suffered an immediate, ugly demise. Our periods of crisis are nowhere near so brief. Whether we're troubled by traffic jams, credit card debts or job insecurity, our bodies assume that we're back in the primeval forest and need to take some form of vigorous action. To prepare us for these crisis situations our brains send out signals which flood our bloodstreams with cholesterol and other high energy fats and sugars. This is generally a totally useless response, since the stressors we meet today can rarely be overcome by any 'fight or flight' reaction.

Nowadays we're constantly being warned of the dangers of eating cholesterol-rich foods, but rarely ever told that cholesterol is a vital component of every cell membrane. Without it, the one million cells which are estimated to die in our bodies every *second* could not be replaced. It's also an essential precursor of all the body's steroid hormones, and plays a crucial role in the creation of the fat soluble vitamins. In addition, it's the main organic molecule in the brain, constituting over half of the dry weight of the cerebral cortex. To safeguard its supply during times of food shortage, every cell in the body has the ability to manufacture cholesterol. This is especially true of the liver, which is the source of about a quarter of the body's endogenous production of cholesterol. When we're under stress, even if we're struggling to follow a fat reduced diet, our blood will be flooded with self-generated cholesterol. This was shown when blood was taken from drivers about to compete in Formula One races. The samples often had a milky white appearance because of their high content of fat. If that fat is not burned up in some form of purposeful activity it will be transferred to the body's fat stores for future use.

This is why stress can make you feel hungry even when you've just eaten. This has been a constant problem for Lord Sugar, who's now reinvented himself as a TV personality since selling his electronic goods company to BSkyB. Prior to that, he'd had a roller-coaster business life, making and losing millions during a career which he admits was at times 'a bloody nightmare'. When interviewed recently he still showed signs of his stressful lifestyle. At the front of his desk he had a mass of biscuits and sweets, which prompted the reporter to ask if he had any favourite comfort foods. 'Oh yeah, yeah,' he replied, 'a lot of people say that when they've got aggravation and trouble they can't eat. It's the complete opposite to me. If something annoying happens, I'll eat, eat, eat.' That's a common reaction today, one survey of a group of five hundred overweight people showing that nearly three-quarters of them ate more when they were worried or nervous, than they did when they were relaxed. (What a pity they couldn't find solace by chewing gum.) A similar response is shown by laboratory animals, as researchers at Pittsburgh University revealed when they subjected two groups of rats to the stress of having their tails pinched at regular intervals. One group served as controls, while the others were given unlimited supplies of sweetened milk. The results showed that after five days, those given the sweet drink option doubled their average calorie intake, gained weight and became significantly heavier than the controls. 'I believe that human beings show tail-pinching behaviour all the time,' was the conclusion the researchers reached. Eating in response to stress is clearly an in-built reaction shown by all animal species, but in humans it's also a conditioned response. It arises when babies discover that solace can be derived from suckling at their mother's breast. In later life, during times of stress, we try to recapture this comforting sensation, a reaction now being exploited by the makers of sweetened milk shakes, one of whom confessed: 'If I could put a nipple on it, I'd be a millionaire.' Many lonely people use eating as a substitute for love, while those with partners recognize that they satisfy this infantile need whenever they refer to them by pet names like sugar, honey and sweetheart.

You'll find that by building a sustaining sexual partnership, and maintaining a network of close, supportive friends, you'll lessen your need to comfort eat. Further help will come from taking firm control of the messages your brain receives. We're information-processing animals, and make judgements based on the data received through our eyes and ears. Before the advent of radio and television signals of distress had a purely parochial distribution. Throughout an entire lifetime a villager might have been involved in only a handful of serious accidents, a few pub brawls, an odd suicide and maybe one or two local murders. Now we live in a global village where death and disaster is our daily fare. This can have a depressing effect, as was shown in Detroit, when a ten-month newspaper strike led to a twenty per cent fall in the local suicide rates. So choose your news input with care, following St Paul's advice to concentrate mainly on those things which are lovely and of good report.

Try to reshape your personal lifestyle so you escape the pressures of 'hurry sickness'. Develop a more relaxed lifestyle. School yourself to cease to worry over petty problems. Adopt the Spanish outlook of *che sera, sera*, or what will be, will be. Don't sweat the small stuff, and remember that it's all small stuff. Develop a proper balance between work and play and discover that what can't be done today can invariably be done tomorrow, or may not need to be done at all. When you find yourself in an angry mood, try to take some form of physical activity to help you work off the stress changes in your body. Any form of abreaction – beating cushions or felling trees – will help relax the tension in your muscles and burn up some of the surplus fats circulating in your bloodstream. To support this change in lifestyle, set aside a few minutes every day for silent meditation. Still your body and you'll immediately calm your mind. Breathe slowly, deeply and gently. Cease to be aware of the passage of time, and enjoy the existential delight of being alive in the here-and-now, so that you come to experience a sense of oneness with the cosmic whole. Remember you are what you eat, but even more so you are what's eating you. Eating doesn't solve problems, it multiplies them.

STEP 29
Learn the art of stress management and you'll reduce your tendency to comfort eat.

STEP 30

Ends are Shaped
by Their Beginnings

We're now coming to the last few weeks of the EssVee programme, which means it's an appropriate time to pause, and pat yourself on the back for what you've achieved so far. It's also an opportunity to recap on some of the steps we've covered so far, to show how they all dovetail together. In Step 11 we stressed the benefits to be gained from eating in a more leisurely fashion, and in Step 24 we recommended that you should slake your thirst before you satisfied your hunger. This week we're building on these two habit changes, which by now should be incorporated in your new, dynamogenic lifestyle. Those earlier assignments provided evidence which showed that people who eat quickly treble their risk of becoming obese. One way of slowing down is to adopt the European custom of starting each meal with a relaxing aperitif. Some people claim that this custom began when a French chemist, by the name of Joseph Dubonnet, set out to create a drink which provided protection against malaria. Its basic active ingredient was quinine, to which he added a selection of medicinal herbs to stimulate the digestion and mask the quinine's bitter taste. This was so tasty that the drink, which was given his name, became a popular aperitif along with Martini and Sherry. Since these pre-dinner drinks are generally served with nibbles – nuts, crackers and olives – they slow us down and give our appestats an early warning that calories are being taken on board.

The same effect is achieved by prefacing a meal by eating portions of fruit. Many people are convinced that they've shed unwanted weight by going on a Grapefruit diet. This has been one of the most popular diets of recent decades, and was put to the test in 2004 at the Nutrition and Metabolic Research Center at Scripps Clinic, San Diego. This trial took a hundred obese adults and divided them into two groups, both of which were encouraged to make a slight increase in their exercise levels. The first group ate three calorie-controlled meals and acted as controls. The other consumed the identical meals, but in their case ate half a grapefruit as a starter course. The results showed that after three months the control group had lost just half a pound, probably because of their increased activity levels, whereas the second had lost an average of over three pounds. The result has been queried, since it was funded by the Florida Citrus Department, but it seems convincing since the subjects taking the grapefruit also showed a reduction in their blood levels of glucose and insulin, which would have made them less prone to develop type 2 diabetes. There is also independent evidence, derived from animal experiments, which shows that grapefruits, and other citrus fruits, contain a flavonoid called naringenin, which makes the liver burn fat instead of sending it for storage.

If you don't fancy eating grapefruits, follow the older, and more widespread, practice of prefacing a meal by eating some form of 'finger food'. This will also send a wake-up call to the brain's satiety centres to let it know that food is being consumed. Most nations have their own speciality dishes. The Italians slake their appetites by eating antipasto, the Chinese put their trust in dim sum, the Russians *zakuski*, the Arabs *meze*, the Japanese sushi and the Swedes smorgasbord. Perhaps the most famous of these starter dishes is the tapas, eaten mainly in Spanish-speaking countries. Originally the tapa was simply a piece of bread put on top of a wine glass to ward off flies and ease the drinker's hunger pangs. In France the equivalent starter dishes are known either as canapés or hors d'oeuvres. The first term means 'couch foods', to signify that they're not eaten at a dining table, while the literal translation of the second term is 'outside of work', which acknowledges that they're appetizers and not part of the main meal.

This is a custom well worth incorporating into your dietary routine. It's a habit that helped to keep our ancestors slim, before the arrival of hurry sickness, fast foods and distracted eating. Add a leisurely course at the start of your meals – an aperitif and olives, a grapefruit segment or any of the multitude of appetizing finger foods – and you'll have less urge to swallow a final course of calorie-rich sweets and puddings.

STEP 30
Make a relaxed start to every main meal by enjoying a leisurely aperitif and maybe some form of tasty tapas or hors d'oeuvres.

STEP 31

Back to the Beginning

Our lifestyle today bears no resemblance to that of our primeval ancestors, and yet there's been no basic change in the way our bodies work since we moved from caves to condominiums. According to scientists working in the field of evolutionary medicine, we haven't yet had time to adjust to the artificial conditions in which we now live. This failure of adaptation is a prime cause of obesity, according to these experts, who believe that our health would improve if we reverted to eating what they describe as a Stone Age diet. This was the fare our forebears ate throughout the entire Paleolithic period, a diet rich in proteins – meat, fish and eggs – accompanied by a wide variety of vegetables, fruits and nuts.

One of the earliest advocates of the Paleolithic diet was Dr Herman Tarnower, a cardiologist who had a fashionable practice in the Scarsdale area of New York. He'd been advising his patients to eat a diet rich in protein but low in fats and sugars, to help them lose weight and lessen their risk of further heart problems. This was so successful that his friends and grateful patients pressed him to write a book setting out his ideas. This he finally did, and the guide which he called *The Complete Scarsdale Medical Diet* immediately entered the best-seller list. It enjoyed a further boost in sales two years later when Dr Tarnower was murdered by his long-term lover, the headmistress of a fashionable boarding school for high school girls in McLeary, Virginia. The Scarsdale diet is now largely forgotten, although it's still recommended by a handful of doctors because it brings about a fairly rapid and dramatic weight loss. This it achieves, partly because it involves a hefty reduction in calorie intake, but more especially because it causes the body to lose large amounts of water. This occurs because protein molecules contain large amounts of nitrogen, unlike molecules of fats and carbohydrates which are made up solely of atoms of carbon, hydrogen and oxygen. Now nitrogen is voided from the body in the form of urea and its breakdown product ammonia, which the kidneys can only discharge in large quantities of water. This explains the sudden weight loss. Unfortunately, like all other crash dieting programmes, the unbalanced Scarsdale regime works only as long as it can be endured. The moment a normal pattern of eating is resumed, the weight which dropped off so rapidly comes piling back with equal speed. (Since urine has a high content of nitrogen, it makes an excellent fertilizer for the roses and runner beans provided it's well diluted with water in a ratio of roughly 8:1.)

Despite these criticisms, there's still much to be said for adopting a Stone Age diet rich in meat, fish and eggs, for proteins are absolutely vital for the maintenance of human health. Every muscle fibre in the body, including those of the vital internal organs, is made up of the protein myosin. Many of the most essential body chemicals – such as insulin and haemoglobin – are proteins. So too are the antibodies which form the foundation of our immune system, and likewise the enzymes which catalyse some four thousand of the body's most crucial chemical reactions. In addition, proteins serve another invaluable function which is often overlooked. They help to stop us gaining excess weight.

This slimming effect arises for two main reasons. In the first place proteins help to trigger a feeling of satiety. Weight for weight they contain less than half as many calories as fats, a gram of fat supplying nine calories, a gram of proteins only four calories. Secondly, and of far greater significance, they trigger what is known as a Specific Dynamic Action (SDA) whenever they're consumed. It takes energy to digest, absorb, metabolize and excrete the food we eat. In the case of proteins, as distinct from carbohydrates and fats, this is a labour-intensive process, since proteins are particularly complex compounds. They're made up of combinations of amino acids, and have to be broken down into these basic building blocks in the intestines before they can be absorbed. Once in the bloodstream they're taken around the body to the cells, where they have to be converted back into proteins. This is a high-energy activity, which generates heat and causes a significant boost in the body's metabolic rate. This is the essence of the SDA, which applies to proteins but to a far lesser extent to fats and carbohydrates. It's often said that weight can be lost by munching a stick of celery, since the energy needed for its digestion exceeds its total calorie content, which is roughly ten calories a stalk. Whether or not this folk tale is true, and it's never been subjected to scientific scrutiny, there's ample proof that eating protein foods triggers a vigorous SDA, an effect which can last for up to fourteen hours. Even when the individual amino acids are surplus to requirements, they still take a larger than average amount of energy to convert them into storable fat – in fact nearly four times as much as when the surplus calories are supplied in the form of fats. So by reverting to a Stone Age diet, and enjoying tasty samples of Tournedos of Filet Mignon Cordon Bleu, we can tickle our taste buds and at the same time keep the excess flab at bay by drawing on the long-lasting metabolic stimulus of the SDA. And if we lack the time for haute cuisine, we can always enjoy the flavour of a lightly boiled egg, which is rich in protein and contains all eight of the essential amino acids, which gain their name because they can't be synthesized within the body.

STEP 31
Reduce your intake of twentieth-century processed food, and return to eating a Stone Age diet rich in proteins, fruit and vegetables.

STEP 32

Master the Art of Gourmet Eating

Once again I make no apology for revisiting some of the ground we've already covered. In doing so I'll quote, by way of justification, the sage words of Dr Samuel Johnston who said, 'men more frequently require to be reminded than informed'. The objective once again is to link up all the individual assignments into one closely woven programme of lifestyle change. So this week we'll link two previous recommendations: don't hurry your pattern of eating, and extract the maximum possible pleasure from the food you eat.

When wine connoisseurs sample a glass of wine they never hurry. To enhance the experience, they hold the glass up to the light to judge the clarity and general appearance of its contents. Once that's done, they'll swill the wine around the glass to release its fragrance and enjoy its 'nose'. Finally, they take a small sample in their mouth so they can savour what sommeliers call its 'in mouth' sensation. If that process is necessary to appreciate a mouthful of wine, it must be still more important to derive the full delight of a mouthful of food, which varies far more in its texture and taste. If we bolt our food, we give it no time to stimulate the fifteen million olfactory receptors which line our mouths. Nature makes sure that activities which are essential for the perpetuation of the species are intensely pleasurable. This applies to sex, and should also pertain to eating.

Nowadays the vogue is for multitasking. People pride themselves on their ability to juggle with several activities at a time, but research in recent years has shown that this can't be done without a loss of efficacy. For instance, students who multitask have been found to suffer more problems with their academic work. Every time they switch their attention from their studies, to receive a text message or change the track on their CD player, their brains have to refocus on the task in hand. Errors creep in and concentration suffers. The same applies to eating. This is one of life's supreme delights which can only be enjoyed to the utmost when we give it our full attention. This doesn't happen when we have our meals while watching TV, reading a book or taking a call on a mobile phone. Every meal should be taken with the concentration that Zen Buddhists show when performing the Japanese Tea Ceremony. As far as possible, eating should be separated from all other behaviours. If not, there's a risk that food will be shovelled down our gullets in an unthinking, indiscriminate manner. The focus should be on the 'here and now', for only then do we maximize our pleasure and give our appestats a chance to tell us when we've had enough. This is also an aid to relaxation, for the more you concentrate on what you're eating, the less you'll fret about the things which are eating you.

Some people graze in a mindless fashion, which means they don't pick up the signals sent by the homeostatic centres in their brain telling them that they've reached the point of satiation. This has been revealed by research work carried out by Dr Marion Hetherington, Professor of Biopsychology at Scotland's Glasgow Caledonian University, who has made a specialist study of appetite regulation. She and her research team have filmed people eating food in a variety of different situations, and discovered that those who fail to focus on what they're doing, and don't notice the taste and smell of their food, will reach the point of satiation far slower than those who do. In some cases this increased their food consumption by as much as thirty per cent. Even watching TV while eating lunch was enough to boost their calorie intake by a not inconsiderable fourteen per cent. This means that anyone who eats two main meals a day can easily consume two hundred calories more than they need simply because of their lack of wholehearted concentration. As a result they'll decrease their enjoyment and at the same time boost their weight by roughly a pound of excess fat every seventeen days. This was the conclusion of Professor Hetherington, who said: 'We believe that focusing on food during eating enhances satiation by facilitating attention and maximizing enjoyment.' Clearly we must train ourselves to be gourmets rather than gourmands. Besides, if we are what we eat, and we're not aware of what we're eating, how do we know who we are?

> ### STEP 32
> Join the ranks of the bon viveurs, and at mealtimes don't multitask but focus your entire attention on the pleasures of eating.

STEP 33

Tiredness Can Kill, and Not Only on the Roads

Obesity is a multi-factorial problem. In essence it may be a case of taking too many calories in and giving too few out, but this imbalance arises for a multitude of different reasons. Unlike the epidemics caused by a specific bacteria or virus, the obesity plague is a hydra-headed fiend. No two people are overweight for exactly the same reasons, some of which are wholly unexpected and may run counter to common sense. For centuries people watched the sun in its daily orbit across the heavens, and had not a moment's doubt that the sun orbited around the earth. That view was shattered by Copernicus who proved that the earth was in fact a satellite of the sun. Doctors are now having to make a similar volte-face. For years it's been generally accepted that fat people lead somewhat dozy lives. The popular idea has been that they put on weight because they're lethargic and as a consequence are always nodding off to sleep. This is what one would expect, since we burn up far fewer calories when we're asleep than when we're up and running. The only sleeping problems that fat people were thought to suffer – like sleep apnoea and a heightened tendency to snore – were thought to be the direct result of their flabby torsos. Now we've got to take on board the recent discovery that many people put on weight, not because they sleep too *much*, but because they sleep too *little*. Needless to say this counter-intuitive concept has not yet featured in any of the standard dietary manuals, but it's a fact that must be included in our EssVee programme. Who knows, maybe the Big Apple has a higher proportion of fatties because New York is a city that never sleeps.

The first inklings of this possibility came in the late 1980s, when a study of 18,000 adults participating in the US government's National Health and Nutrition Examination Survey revealed that those who got less than six hours' sleep a night had a twenty-three per cent higher risk of being obese than those who got the recommended seven hours or more. The risk shot up to fifty per cent for those who were unmitigated sleep cheats and got less than five hours' sleep a night. Subsequent research has now verified this chance observation. Scientists at Wake Forest University, California, have monitored a thousand Americans with a high risk of developing obesity-related disorders, and found that those under forty who regularly get less than five hours' sleep a night gain an average of three pounds more than those who sleep for six or seven hours. They also discovered that it's possible to have too much of a good thing, for the layabouts in their sample who regularly slept for more than eight hours a night gained nearly two pounds more than those who kept to the recommended level of six or seven. When CAT scans were taken, it was found that most of the excess fat was laid down around the belly and visceral organs, which makes it particularly liable to cause serious complications.

Subsequent studies of over a thousand volunteers, carried out by researchers at the University of Bristol in the UK, and Stanford University in America, have revealed that compared with people who sleep for less than five hours a night, those who sleep for two hours more show a fifteen per cent lower level of ghrelin in their bloodstream. This is the hormone generated in the stomach which sends hunger messages to the brain to signal that it's time to eat. They also showed a reduction in their metabolic rate, and a fifteen per cent fall in their circulatory levels of leptin, the naturally occurring hormone produced in the fat cells, which registers a lack of stored energy and triggers an increased desire to eat. All three of these biological changes mean that after a night with too little sleep, people may well be too tired to exercise, yet feel a compulsion to consume high energy food and drinks.

This is a particular problem for children today when so many of them are allowed to stay up late, watching TV or playing computer games in their bedroom. A longitudinal study of thirteen thousand British children, carried out in conjunction with the Avon Longitudinal Study of Parents and Children, revealed that those who were poor sleepers at thirty months were more likely to be obese by the time they reached the age of seven. In the words of one of the research team: 'Earlier bed times, later wake times and later school start times could be an important and relatively low-cost strategy to help reduce childhood weight problems ... We found even an hour of sleep makes a big difference.'

Those who find it difficult to conjure up the muse of sleep may find it helpful to take a late-night stroll before retiring to bed. This is the recipe recommended by Benjamin Franklin, who observed: 'Fatigue is the best pillow.' Far better to exercise last thing at night, than eat. Anyone who gets their recommended ration of sleep will not only reduce their weight problems, but also derive a number of spin-off benefits. The average amount of sleep required by over-weight people may well be two hours more. Those who get this allowance will reduce their risk of hypertension, and also improve their appearance. Far better the benison of sleep to keep the wrinkles at bay than six-monthly shots of Botox. This was shown recently when Swedish researchers photographed the faces of twenty-three young adults after a normal night's sleep, and then again after a period of enforced sleep reduction. When a panel of observers was asked to assess the photographs, they had no difficulty recognizing that the sleep deprived were more tired, but they also judged them to be less healthy and attractive. A tired look is an old look, and we need our beauty sleep to enhance our appearance, and also, we now know, to keep us slim.

STEP 33
Make sure you get a good night's sleep, for this will reduce your risk of putting on weight, and improve your general well-being.

STEP 34

Self-esteem:
The Perfect Pick-me-up

By now the *lietmotif* of this book should be as clear as a mountain stream. Obesity is a lifestyle disorder and not a straightforward medical disease like measles or ingrowing toenails. It's our outlook and way of life that matters, and not just the amount and quality of the food we eat. This was revealed when a study was made of the health and mental attitude of a group of 6,500 ten-year-old children, carried out in 1970 by a research team from King's College, London. When the children were followed up twenty years later, it was found that those who originally showed low self-esteem, and felt they had scant control of their destinies, were significantly more likely to develop into obese adults. This outcome, which applied more closely to girls than to boys, suggests that it's low self-esteem that makes us fat, rather than the other way around. The more you learn to like yourself, the more you'll treasure your appearance and physical fitness. Don't waste time focusing on your faults, spend it boosting your attributes. After all, you spend more time with yourself than with anyone else, so you may as well make sure you enjoy these encounters.

Why do we allow ourselves to become the victims of this tragic self-neglect? Men nowadays will run up hefty credit card debts to pay for hair transplants and cosmetic surgery, while their partners will regularly spend a small fortune on cosmetics and hair-dos. Yet, despite making these narcissistic gestures, a high percentage of people in the developed countries will allow their bodies to grow dysfunctional and misshapen. Some think that this is an act of God, an event which is totally beyond their control. That's why at the start of the programme we asked you to explore the relevance of Professor Julian Rotter's 'locus of control' theory. This challenges us to accept that the success or failure of our lives – and our chance of achieving lifetime weight control – lies in our own hands. You, dear reader, and you alone are the master of your fate and the captain of your soul. Another psychological defence mechanism, commonly used by long-term members of the Corpulent Club, is to deny that they are in fact overweight. To make it difficult for you to sustain that myth, we asked you to stand in the nude and eye your figure in front of a full-length bathroom mirror. By now, if you've been diligent in your pursuit of your weekly assignments, you'll be in far better shape. So it's a good time to take another peer into the glass and see what you've achieved. Give yourself a congratulatory pat on the back for the pounds you've lost, and maybe a stimulatory slap on the rump to remind you of the work you've still to do. That can be judged by submitting yourself to the pinch test. Grip the skin midway between your navel and groin with your thumb and forefinger. Then measure the size of the fold you've grasped. If you're a man, you're carrying excess fat if the fold measures more than nineteen millimetres, which is roughly the thickness of your little finger. If you're a woman, the fold should measure no more than twenty-seven millimetres, which is the thickness of the average woman's thumb. Any thicker than this, and you've still more weight to lose.

One way of speeding your progress is to focus on boosting your self-esteem. Our personal appearance is one of the things which does most to give us a sense of justifiable pride. This isn't preening, it's a process which adds to our feeling of efficacy and self-worth. There's often a dangerous gap between the person we are, and the person we'd like to be. The wider that rift, the more dissatisfied we become. This creates a vicious circle, for the lower our self-esteem, the more depressed we become and the greater our inertia and tendency to overeat. Recent research shows that there are one or two relatively simple things that can be done to gain a psychological fillip. One earlier assignment was to carry out muscle-building activities. This is a wise policy because, weight for weight, skeletal muscles consume nearly three times more energy than fat, even when they're totally at rest. This means that the more muscles you develop and maintain, the easier you'll find it to stay slim. The bonus, it's recently been discovered, is that having a tight, muscular figure will also contribute in no small measure to your overall self-esteem. This was shown when Aaron Lukaszeweski, a researcher at the University of California, measured the strength of 174 students and found that those who were physically strong were much more self-assured and outward going than those with less muscular frames. This one factor accounted for thirty per cent of the difference found, which Lukaszeweski asserts is 'a huge effect for something as nebulous as personality'. Posture is another factor which contributes to self-esteem. It's never difficult to spot the members of a losing side at the end of a gruelling football match. They walk with downcast eyes, whereas the heads of the champions are held aloft in triumph. It's useful to harness this response, because your mood can be changed by altering the carriage of your head and modifying the direction of your gaze. Psychological studies have been carried out in which volunteers were given the simple task of moving marbles, either downwards or upwards. The results showed that when the marbles were moved to a higher level, the subjects were more likely to recall positive memories from the day before than when they were moving them downwards. This suggests that we can boost our mood simply by modifying the tilt of our head. Something similar was found by two psychologists at Northwestern University, Illinois, who tested seventy-seven students and found that when they adopted a confident, dominant posture they felt a sense of power which was twenty-four per cent greater than when they sat in a constricted, hunched posture. So hold yourself in a way which conveys your feeling of quiet confidence and control. Boost your self-esteem, and generate an uplifting, on-top-of-the-world sensation, by imagining that you're a puppet being lifted up by its central string.

We need to boost our self-esteem, for this is a sign not of vanity but of inner strength. Work to achieve your full potential. Cultivate self-respect, and then you'll be less likely to sink into a state of disrepair. Learn to love yourself, bearing in mind the advice that the Buddha gave his disciples: 'You yourself, as much as anybody else in the entire universe, deserve your love and affection.'

STEP 34
Boost your self-esteem, and you'll have far less risk of having a surfeit of fat or a dearth of confidence.

STEP 35

Don't be a Hoarder or Shopaholic

Where did it all go wrong? Our forebears were nomads, and over thousands of years evolved in a way which enabled them to carry stores of food, not in their arms or on their backs, which would have impeded their movements, but in a network of fat stores carried within their own bodies. That's a system we're still using today, even though we now follow a vastly different way of life, and generally live within a few minutes' drive of a well-stocked food store. What's more, why do we think we have to ape the habits of hamsters, who are schooled from birth to maintain a cache of food within easy reach of their nests? Like these humble rodents, we've become inveterate food hoarders. (The word hamster comes from the German *hamstern* meaning 'to hoard'.) Squirrels do something similar, although they scatter their food stores in several different locations to reduce the risk of pilfering. We've stupidly chosen to adopt the same practice, scattering our personal space with hidden food reserves, carried in our cars, pockets, pantries, larders, fridges and office desks. Yet nobody can steal our fat stores, or at least they couldn't until plastic surgeons developed the technique of liposuction. In today's world we have no need whatsoever to pursue the risky practice of hoarding food.

If we're constantly surrounded by stores of food, the temptation to overeat is greatly increased. When food is within easy reach, it's all too easy to nibble mindlessly while watching TV or sitting behind the wheel of a car. Just as people often refuse to believe they're overweight, so many find it difficult to acknowledge the actual amount of food they consume. One way to overcome this delusion is to keep a diary record of every morsel of food you eat. This is an effective exercise which we advise you to try this week, and at odd times in the future, because the mere fact of having to keep an honest record of every biscuit or chocolate that enters your mouth is generally enough to reduce your overall food consumption. This was shown when a study was made of 1,700 overweight patients attending the Kaiser Permanente Center for Health Research at Oregon. All the participants were placed on the same weight-reducing diet, but half were given the additional task of recording everything they ate. The results showed that those who kept the diary record lost an average of almost eighteen pounds in six months, compared with the control group, who dieted but didn't keep the diary record, who lost an average of just nine pounds.

Another way of overcoming the hoarding habit is to take special care when entering food stores. Overeating is an addiction, which supermarkets are eager to foster, so don't be lured by their tempting offers. Studies have shown that overweight people are particularly sensitive to the sight, smell and availability of food, which means the more often they go to food stores, the more they're tempted to buy. So aim to cut down your visits to supermarkets, if possible to a maximum of one a week. Draw up a shopping list before you cross their threshold, and refuse every enticement to impulse buy. Make substitutions if necessary, but don't buy anything that's not on your predetermined list. If you haven't tabled it, you don't need it. Be aware too of the marketing tricks that food suppliers use. Supermarkets know that by positioning food in certain places – particularly at the end of the aisle or by the checkout counter – they can achieve a five-fold increase in impulse buying. So exercise particular care at the checkout, where the stores display high-profit items which are generally low in nutritional values. Don't buy ready-prepared meals, only foods that require your loving care and painstaking preparation. And don't fill your trolley to earn extra bonus points on your loyalty card, which is rather like giving children a sweetie if they clear up their toys before they go to bed.

Buy what you want to eat, not what the store wants to sell. If you're a sucker when exposed to the sight and smell of food, adopt the policy of the British prime minister Harold Wilson, who told a journalist that he always did his food shopping after he'd had a meal and felt replete. Avoid two-for-one offers like the plague. That's the advice given by Catherine Collins, the chief dietitian at St George's Hospital, London, who admits: 'I caught myself buying two packets of biscuits at a time thinking they would last longer. Actually I just ate more biscuits.' Experiments show that we always increase our level of consumption when food is served in large containers, so if it's economical to buy the super-market's jumbo-sized packs of biscuits and breakfast cereals, make sure you transfer them into smaller boxes the moment you return home. Don't be lured by press reports of food shortages and pending price rises, which always result in panic buying. And don't buy a fridge that is larger than you need because, whatever its size, the tendency will always be to fill it to the brim, to create a feeling of security and affluence. Many people will store food in their fridge even though it's long past its sell-by date. This satisfies their hoarding instinct, and helps conceal the fact that they've over purchased. To overcome this wasteful habit, make a strict point of clearing your fridge every month.

> **STEP 35**
> Don't hoard, or over source, food, which is fine for hamsters but potentially lethal for humans.

STEP 36

Pumping the Bellows and Fanning the Internal Fires

Life on earth couldn't exist without a never-ending supply of oxygen. From the instant we're born and take our first, faltering gasp, to the moment we die and utter our final, departing sigh, our lives are dependent on this life-sustaining element. This was recognized by the ancient Roman sages, who used the same word, '*spiritus*' to describe both 'breath' and 'life force'. Our mood, our energy levels, our stamina and longevity all depend on the efficiency of our respiratory systems. Nowadays we're obsessed with food, yet humans can go for weeks without food but can survive only minutes without air. Every day we need to absorb about thirty-five pounds of air, which is six times our daily consumption of food and drink. And the miracle is that this vital fuel is totally free and in unlimited supply. Some snake oil salesmen are now pedalling 'personal oxygen generators', to replace what they claim is a lack of oxygen in the air over many industrial cities. As part of their pitch they assert that the oxygen concentration of the air over Tokyo has dropped to a perilous five per cent. This is utter poppycock, for throughout the globe the level of atmospheric oxygen remains at a steady twenty-one per cent as it has been since human life began. Even if we went on burning billions of tons of fossil fuels for the next few decades the present levels of oxygen would only fall by one per cent, which is far less than the drop we experience on days when the barometric pressure falls, or we climb a hill one hundred metres high.

Many people today are suffering breathing problems, but at normal ground levels this can never be attributed to a shortage of oxygen in the air. The fault invariably lies with our personal breathing apparatus. Either we've got problems with our cardiopulmonary systems, in which case we should consult a doctor, or we're in poor physical condition, in which case we should take immediate steps to get ourselves fit. We shouldn't be short of puff when we climb a flight of stairs. This is a useful test for couch potatoes, for while you can lie about your age, you can't cheat a flight of stairs. Another handy check is to take the Sabrazés Test, which was developed at the very start of the twentieth century by Dr Jean Sabrazés, a French physician who noted that patients who have difficulty holding their breath are poor operative risks. To carry out this simple fitness test, exhale as fully as you can and then see how long you can last without having to take another breath. If you're a male, you should be able to hold out for at least thirty seconds; for women the target is twenty seconds or more. If you're an athlete, you should be able to do far better than this, for in 2009 a Hungarian deep sea diver set a world record when he stayed immersed for twenty-one minutes!

One of the most important measures of physical fitness is the vital capacity of our lungs. A large study carried by the Health Research Trust, Cambridge, showed that a poor chest capacity was the most outstanding feature of people with poor general health. Another research project followed up a group of well over a thousand senior citizens for five years. This revealed that the most accurate predictor of five-year survival was the individual's peak expiratory flow rate, which is a measure of the power with which the lungs can expel air. Medical researchers agree that breathing is one of the fundamental secrets of longevity. All you've got to do is keep it up for a hundred years! The average sedentary worker today uses only about a tenth of their total lung capacity, and there's a very real risk that they'll suffer a significant decline in lung function if the remaining nine-tenths is not brought into play from time to time. This hazard is magnified if they happen to be not only inactive but also overweight. When we inspire, about sixty per cent of the space needed for the expansion of our lungs comes from the descent of the diaphragm. The piston-like action of this large sheet of muscle is hampered if the abdominal organs and belly wall are laden with fat. Prolonged mental tension can have also have a strait-lacing effect. Most emotional states are accompanied by changes in our pattern of breathing. We gasp with alarm, catch our breath when we're afraid, yawn when we're bored and groan when we're upset. If we want to hide our emotions, as we often do in today's tight-lipped society, we can only do so by keeping a tight check on our breathing. Everything nowadays conspires to restrict our intake of oxygen, and this can make it extra hard to lose weight.

It's easy to forget that our bodies are highly complex metabolic factories, which constantly carry out several thousand separate oxidative processes. Every one of these activities burns up calories and consumes oxygen. When slimmers set out to burn up calories, they instantly think of taking strenuous physical exercise; in fact, sixty per cent of the calories we consume goes on maintaining our internal chemical processes. If we don't ensure an adequate intake of oxygen, our metabolic fires will be damped down and the unburned fuel transported to our fat stores. This means there's a very close link between breathing and weight control. Every breath we take consumes one watt of energy. This was once one of the favourite slimming techniques used at the prestigious Walke Sanatorium in Wiesbaden, Germany, where it was found that many overweight people breathe badly and can be helped to regain a normal weight balance by carrying out a regular series of deep breathing exercises. A similar technique is employed by Vyasa International, a yoga movement which runs a slimming clinic at its headquarters in Bangalore. Here the overweight are taught to close their left nostril and breathe rapidly through their right nostril exactly twenty-seven times. This practice – which has to be repeated four times daily prior to meals and before retiring to bed – is claimed to boost the body's metabolic rate and lead to a typical weight loss of two kilograms a week. This is impossible to believe, and I'd advise you to put your faith in the technique employed by Dame Eva Turner, the world-famous opera singer. Throughout her life she made a practice of going for a brisk walk during which she inhaled for twelve strides, held her breath for twelve strides and then exhaled for the next dozen paces. You may not be able to do this to begin with, but with regular practice your performance will show a slow but steady step-by-step improvement. It certainly kept Dame Eva on song, and helped her live well into her hundredth year. By her example she proved the truth of the old Sanskrit maxim: 'He who only half breathes, only half lives.'

STEP 36

Give a boost to your energy output, and shed more surplus weight, by stepping up your intake of oxygen-rich air.

STEP 37

Mind Over Platter

It's all too easy to think of obesity as a purely physical problem, a one-eyed approach which totally ignores the influence of the mind. You're not what you think you are, but what you think, you are. Juvenal, the Roman satirist, was right on the button when he introduced the concept of *mens sana in corpore sano*, for it's only when we establish a healthy outlook of mind that we can hope to develop a truly healthy body. If we harness the powers of our mind, we'll have no need to eat special foods, pump iron, count calories or read endless weight-loss books. Inside our skulls we all have a computer which is infinitely more powerful than any we could buy in a high street store. Anyone who harnesses the might of this cybernetic masterpiece will be well on the way to achieving their health goals. This needs to be done at two levels.

The first step is to take charge of your subconscious mind, ridding it of any negative thoughts that may be harboured there. Are you secretly clinging on to excuses for not losing weight? Are you still blaming your genes, or your misfortune in having been born to chubby parents? If so, banish these bogus notions from your mind. Whatever your circumstances, nature wants you to be healthy, and you can't achieve that ideal state if you're overweight. Eliminate the negative, and accentuate the positive. Reassure yourself by making a daily affirmation: 'Every day in every way I'm getting slimmer and slimmer.' That was the mantra that Emile Coué, the father of autosuggestion, got his overweight patients to recite when they made a pilgrimage to his famous clinic in the French town of Nancy. Be firm in your resolve. Don't entertain any thoughts of failure. This you can do by reciting another of Coué's favourite avowals, which Barack Obama adopted on his road to the White House: 'I can, I can, I can!' There's no need to call on the help of hypnotists and mind coaches. That's a cop out, which transfers the responsibility from the subject to the therapist, who then gets the blame if the scales fail to budge. This was acknowledged by Coué who said: 'Everyone carries the instrument of their own well-being in their brain. The function of the therapist is merely to help patients adopt an attitude of healthy mindedness.'

But we're ornery critters, which is another thing that Coué's followers discovered. Tell a child to eat their greens and they'll do the exact opposite. In the same way, if adults set out to stop eating sweets, their longing for sweets will strengthen. This is a phenomenon known as 'contrary imagination', which for some reason is stronger in women than in men. According to Mark Twain, when Adam was in the Garden of Eden, 'He did not want the apple for the apple's sake, he wanted it because it was forbidden.' In a recent trial, a team of psychologists took people with a passion for chocolate and divided them into two groups. The subjects in the first group were told to come to terms with their liking for chocolate, while those in the second were asked to put it out of their minds and overcome their yearning. Some time later, when they were given the opportunity of taking their pick from a wide selection of tasty chocolates, it was found that those who'd been told to control their cravings ate fifty per cent more than those who'd been allowed to give free rein to their imagination.

In 1999, readers of the *Daily Telegraph* newspaper were invited to take part in a slimming experiment, supervised by Dr James Levine of the Mayo Clinic, Minnesota. The volunteers were asked to remain on their normal diets, but to follow one of two weight-loss regimes. One option was to step up their general level of exercise, the other to think themselves slimmer, by picturing themselves a few pounds lighter, imagining that they were carrying out strenuous exercise and feeling better about their general image. Over three hundred chose the mind-control routine, over half of whom registered a significant weight loss. But while our unconscious minds have enormous influence, we must also harness the full potential of that part of the brain which is responsible for conscious, rational thought. 'Management by objectives' is a well-established business principle. Whatever you want to achieve, you must have clearly defined goals, and a well-defined route by which those targets can be reached. No one plans to fail, but multitudes fail to plan. When psychologist Peter Gollwitzer of New York University quizzed a group of subjects about their goal-seeking activities, he found that those who went to the trouble of making detailed where-when-and-how plans were about three times as likely to attain their chosen goal. 'Planning can turn a difficult conscious decision into an unconscious habit,' he concluded, which is, of course, the very essence of the EssVee slimming programme.

And there's another good reason why we should make better use of our brains, a biological reality which hasn't been mentioned so far in any of the medical literature I've studied in my researches for this book. The brain comprises only two per cent of the weight of the human body, and yet it consumes twenty per cent of the body's total energy intake. The more it's stimulated – whether by writing poems, playing chess, solving cryptic crosswords or debating with friends – the more energy it consumes. Just like our muscles, our brain cells become flabby if they're under employed. We either 'use them or lose them', and the more we put them to use the more active and exciting our lives become, and the easier it is to keep slim.

STEP 37

Take care to exercise your brain as well as your body. Think yourself slim, and burn up calories by giving your brain a regular work-out.

STEP 38

When a Cow Becomes
a Man's Best Friend

There are times when major medical advances are made, not
by inventing the new, but by rediscovering the old. It's a
process well enshrined in the old French saying '*Reculer pour
mieux sauter*', which roughly translated means 'to step back,
in order to better jump forward'. That's a step we're going
to take this week. Well over a century ago, Dr Philippe
Karell, physician to His Majesty the Emperor of Russia,
published an influential paper entitled 'The Milk Cure'.
This was published in medical journals on both sides of the
Atlantic, and told of the excellent results he'd obtained by
putting obese patients on a regime of three to four glasses of
semi-skimmed milk a day. His general conclusion – that
'milk is the best and surest of remedies' – encouraged many
doctors to put their overweight patients on diets rich in
skimmed milk, cottage cheese and low-fat yoghurts. That
policy was only abandoned in recent years, following the ill-
founded brouhaha about the dangers of eating foods which
were judged to carry too much 'bad' cholesterol. But the tide
is about to turn, for recent research has shown that dairy
foods are not only a vital part of a healthy, balanced diet, but
also serve as a 'superfood' for slimmers.

When I was a lad, dairy foods contributed about seventy
per cent of the average adult's total intake of calcium. In
those days doctors knew that babies were healthier if they
were fed on mother's milk, because it was such a good source
of this vital mineral. Now they also know that breast-fed
babies are less likely to become obese in later life than those
who are weaned too soon on to solid foods. In those enlight-
ened days, youngsters were given free milk at school to aid

the sturdy growth of their bones. That came to an abrupt end when the health police decided that people who consumed dairy foods ran an increased risk of falling victim to heart attacks and strokes. This myth lingers on, even though it doesn't stand up to scientific scrutiny. If there's such a thing as original sin, which I find difficult to believe when I gaze into the face of a newborn babe, it's that we often fail to question the reality of what we're told. As a result we may take years to adopt the truth, but only seconds to accept fallacies and falsehoods. Five years ago a study published in the *Lancet* revealed that there was an inverse relationship between cholesterol levels and heart disease in older people. This completely overthrew the accepted dogma of the day, proving conclusively that the lower a person's blood cholesterol level, the higher their risk of all-cause mortality. This finding was later underpinned by research carried out by Professor Peter Elwood at Cardiff University. He tracked a group of over two thousand men for twenty years and found that those who drank full fat milk, and ate cheese and yoghurt, were less likely to suffer diabetes, heart disease and stroke.

Earlier sections of this book have made regular reference to the appestat, the controlling centre in the brain which regulates our appetite according to our energy needs. At this point I'm going to postulate a far more sophisticated cybernetic system. Here I'm going out on a limb, because I've no proof whatsoever that the system exists, but knowing that man is 'fearfully and wonderfully made', I find it easier to believe that it does, than that it doesn't. Our bodies must have an adequate intake of calcium and other essential nutrients, and it seems reasonable to expect that our bodies must possess a homeostatic mechanism which ensures that we eat enough to meet these requirements. If that supposition is true, there's a very real risk that if we reduce our intake of dairy foods, we may be encouraged to go on eating a wide range of calorie-rich rubbish – chips, hamburgers, cakes, sweets, and doughnuts – until we finally satisfy our vital calcium needs.

In the past several studies have shown a clear link between obesity and low intakes of calcium, but these have been largely ignored by the medical profession because of its reluctance to exorcise the cholesterol bogey. Early experiments with laboratory animals, carried out at the University of Tennessee, showed that increasing the dietary intake of calcium tends to encourage the breakdown of fat, a process known as lipolysis. This almost certainly applies to humans, as was first suggested in a report published in 2001 in the *International Journal of Obesity*, which followed the fortunes of a group of fifty-three children of pre-school age. This revealed that those who had the highest intake of calcium showed the lowest body fat measurements. The same applies to adults, as has been shown by researchers working under the direction of Professor Angelo Tremblay, holder of the Canada Research Chair in Physical Activity, Nutrition and Energy Balance. They found that half the women attending their obesity clinic were living on calcium-deficient diets. Taking a typical group, they discovered that their average intake of calcium was less than 600 mg a day, compared with the Recommended Daily Allowance of 1000 mg. All were placed on the same low-calorie diet, but some were given tablets which supplied them with 1200 mg of calcium a day, while the others received identical looking placebo pills. At the end of the trial it was found that the women taking the calcium supplements had lost nearly six times as much weight as those who took the inert pills.

Prompted by the media, many overweight people are now placing their faith in 'super foods', like grapefruits, berries and green tea, which are rich in antioxidants. These, they're led to believe, will 'melt' away their surplus fat. Dairy foods would seem to be a far better bet. This was confirmed by a follow-up study, also published in the *International Journal of Obesity*, in which obese adults were put on a low-calorie diet and then divided into two groups. One group ate three daily servings of low-fat yoghurt a day, the other consumed just one. All the participants lost significant amounts of fat, while still maintaining their mass of lean muscle tissue, but those taking the three daily servings lost 22 per cent more weight, 61 per cent more body fat, and 81 per cent more stomach fat than those restricted to a single serving. We've long accepted the value of a 'Mediterranean diet', which is generally attributed to its high content of wine, olive oil and fresh vegetables, but it may well be that the benefits are due to the fact that the people of Southern France and Italy have a great love of dairy foods, coupled with their widespread culinary use of butter, cheese and cream. This is certainly the belief of the French Board for Nutrition and Health, which now recommends the consumption of three helpings of dairy food a day for adults, and four helpings for children.

STEP 38
Follow the Karell Cure, and step up your daily intake of calcium-rich dairy products.

STEP 39

Fast and Furious

Congratulations! Now's the time for celebrations, since you've reached the final week of your thirty-nine week EssVee programme. One way to mark this landmark occasion is to go through your wardrobe and throw away all your fat clothes. These you'll never need again. After that, you should mark the event, not by holding a family feast, but by taking a one-day fast. That's an old pagan practice, followed because it produces a feeling of euphoria, similar to that gained by taking LSD or magic mushrooms. (I've never experienced a psychedelic high through fasting, or I'd have done it more often!) Since the advent of monotheistic religions, Jews have taken a day's fast to commemorate the Day of Atonement, and Muslims have abstained from food from dawn to dusk to mark the thirty days of Ramadan. Recent research suggests that, far from having adverse side effects, these short fasts can provide a definite physiological fillip. Some Mormons make a practice of fasting for one day every month, which seems to improve their long-term health, for a recent review of over five hundred elderly patients attending the medical centre at Salt Lake City, Utah, revealed that Mormons who fasted one day a month were 39 per cent more likely to have healthy hearts than those who didn't fast at all.

In view of these potential benefits, it's unfortunate that fasting has been linked with one or two less reputable practices, like 'de-toxification'. In 1977 Dr Goldstein published *Triumph Over Disease*, a book which suggested that fasting was 'the body-cleanser supreme'. This is a complete fallacy, based on the observation that spells of fasting often give rise to bad breath and a coated tongue. These symptoms invariably arise when fats are broken down – as happens when diabetics suffer a spell of hypoglycaemia – and are in no way a sign that the body is being purged of injurious toxins. (The author of the book can be forgiven for making this mistake, for he was a podiatrist and so better qualified to treating hammer toes than sagging jowls and bulging bellies.) The use of fasting as a means of political protest has shown how long people can survive without eating. Gandhi demonstrated this point, although some of his biographers reckon his devotees kept him alive by giving him enemas which, while ostensibly designed to prevent dehydration, also carried significant quantities of glucose and honey. A more credible example is Dick Gregory, the US comedian and TV chat show host. He went on a well-supervised fast to protest against America's involvement in the Vietnam War. It lasted from Thanksgiving Day to New Year's Eve, and while it did little to influence the conduct of the war, it had a dramatic effect on Gregory. He lost several stones, and went from being decidedly plump to becoming trim, slim and far younger looking than his true age. More important, it made a profound and lasting effect on his lifestyle, making him more aware of what he ate, and prompting him to resume the athletic activities he enjoyed so much as a young man.

Bringing about such a lifestyle change can help prolong our lives, as was recognized by the ancient Chinese, who claimed that fasting, which they knew as *p'i ku*, was one of the most important of the 'cordials of immortality'. Laboratory experiments show that the lifespan of mice can be increased some 40 per cent if they're fed for two days and then starved on the following day. So far there's no evidence that the same applies to humans, although many gerontologists are convinced it does. You certainly can't be fit and fat, for if you're obese your chances of contracting fatal heart disease are doubled, you're more likely to have a stroke, and you expose yourself to well over twice the risk of developing type 2 diabetes. In fact, anyone who's overweight is carrying a load of trouble. When men of average build carry twenty pounds of excess flab, they're forced to use fourteen per cent more energy to heave themselves from place to place. This makes them tired and creates a vicious circle, for the quicker their get-up-and-go has got up and gone, the less exercise they're inclined to take. Many people claim that they're sick and tired of being overweight, when what they really mean is that they're sick and tired *through* being overweight.

Dr Sidney Lecker, an American psychiatrist, admits that he's a food junkie 'who must fast in order to maintain a healthy and attractive body'. He makes this confession in his preface to a book on *Fasting*, by Judith Dobrzynski. He's come to realize that he will always have a passion for eating and be what he calls 'a psychologically fat person'. However he's also noted that his appreciation of food is lessened when he eats too much, and claims that: 'Fasting helps us rediscover what good food really tastes like.' This is in line with the old German proverb: 'Fasting today makes the food good tomorrow.' So this week's task is to take a ritual fast as a rite of passage, partly to celebrate your completion of the Slim Vitality course, but more especially to drive away your fear of hunger and demonstrate that you – with the help of your internal appestat – are in total charge of your body. Limit this fast to a single day, otherwise you run the risk of losing vital body tissues. This was shown when a group of seventy men undertook a ten-day fast. During this period they shed an average of well over twenty pounds, but only just over a third of this loss was fat, the remainder consisted of muscle, bone and vital organ tissues. So limit your fast to a single day, during which time you should keep up a high level of physical exercise and drink plenty of water and fruit juices so you don't suffer dehydration. This was the basis of the WOW diet – which stands for **W**alking, **O**ranges and **W**ater – which the media took to be the highlight of my book *Farewell to Fatigue*. If you do this, you'll be following in the footsteps of Sir Francis Chichester, who was an inspiration to the world's golden oldies in 1966 when he set the world speed record for a solo, round-the-world sailing navigation at the remarkable age of sixty-six. To keep himself fit he regularly took a two-day fast, during which he slaked his thirst by drinking only apple juice. Every time he did so he felt stronger, happier, and more full of energy. This he records in his book *How to Keep Fit,* in which he avers, 'for me fasting is the most beneficial treatment I have ever received'. Do this from time to time – when you're free of other chores and can concentrate on the task in hand – and you'll revolutionize your eating habits and lose anything from one to three pounds a time. (**Warning**: Don't do this without consulting your doctor if you have any doubts about your general health or are suffering from diabetes, high blood pressure or coronary disease.)

STEP 39

Readjust your eating habits, and overcome your fear of going hungry, by taking an occasional one-day fast.

Finale

Congratulations on completing the course! You may not yet be down to your desired weight, but that will come providing you continue to pursue your new, dynamogenic lifestyle. As long as you feel good, and look good, there's nothing else to worry about. Keep following the programme, and listening to the wisdom of your body, and you'll soon reach a Body Mass Index which is appropriate for your height, skeletal structure and genetic make-up. From now onwards you must live in the present, learn from the past and prepare for the future The future is not something which is presented to us, it is something we ourselves create. In retrospect, these last nine months will surely be among the most important of your entire life, for during them you've acquired a range of habits which will not only help you maintain a healthy weight, but will also serve to improve your health, lengthen your life, enhance your appearance, boost your energy levels, increase your happiness and swell your circle of friends. That change in lifestyle is also likely to boost your wealth, for surveys show that overweight people consistently earn less than their slim, trim peers. Any extra cash you gain will be an enormous boon, for wealth is now the greatest driver of health outcomes. At one time a gold watch chain, proudly displayed across a bulging belly, was worn by rich landowners and 'bloated' capitalists to display their affluence. Now obesity is the bugbear of the poor, rather than the status symbol of the rich. The latest UK figures show that a twenty-year-old male in social class I can expect to live five years longer than one in social class V. This means it's more important for the community to tackle poverty than to combat cancer, for even if cancer could be totally eradicated, life expectancy would only be extended by three years.

Fat Liberation
Obesity is a personal choice and like all other plagues, it's a communicable disease. This book has been chiefly concerned with the harm it does to individuals, but that's nothing compared with the damage it does to the community at large. In future no government in the world can afford to ignore its insidious effect, for the health, happiness and economic success of a nation can never exceed the sum total of the well-being and working efficiency of its inhabitants. This is a social issue which only communities can solve. Social progress will be made the moment the 'me' generation learns to become the 'we' generation. Movements are now being formed – like the International Size Acceptance Association – which are trying to seize the moral high ground and get us to stop using the abusive F word. They want society to accept overweight people as readily and compassionately as it does dwarves and people born with club feet. As a result of their public agitation they've spun off one or two activist movements, such as Fat Pride, Fat Power and Fat Liberation. Fortunately these provocateur groups have had precious little impact, which is not surprising since they're total misnomers. Nobody who is fat can be proud, powerful or liberated, when they're engulfed in ungainly tyres of roly-poly fat which make them like Michelin cartoon characters. There's ample reason to argue against ageism and sexism, since people are not responsible for their age or sex, but the same can't be said of 'weightism', since this is invariably a self-inflicted illness. Any discrimination against the obese is not based on their bulk, but on their judgement. They have chosen to follow an obesogenic lifestyle, which is not only damaging *their* lives, it's also impairing the welfare of their neighbours, since it gives rise to mounting health care costs and reduced economic productivity. Experts at the London School of Hygiene and Tropical Medicine have recently published a study suggesting that since the obese eat 18 per

cent more than average, they are unfairly contributing to world hunger and rising food prices. To counter these arguments the fat acceptance campaigners have coined a catchy slogan, 'a diet is a cure that doesn't work, for a disease that doesn't exist'. That's a typically one-eyed statement, for while they're undoubtedly right that crash dieting rarely results in any long-term good, it's totally false to suggest that obesity is not a bona fide ailment. The last thing we should do is make it socially acceptable, for then it will make sufferers less likely to amend their ways. Instead of treating obesity as the norm, we must henceforth regard it is an unacceptable aberration. As with smoking, it must in future become just as socially unacceptable to display overweight bodies in public, as it is to spit or walk about with unkempt hair, halitosis and filthy nails.

Catalysts for Change

A parent's job is to protect their children from long-term harm, which means helping them adopt a healthy lifestyle so that when they mature they'll no longer need the protection of their parents, or the support of a nanny state's welfare benefits and medical services. If we see children at risk when they're playing with fireworks, we intervene and urge them to take care. We should have the courage to do exactly the same when our family and friends are putting on weight, for they too are playing with fire. If you've benefited by following the EssVee programme, please spread the good news. At this very moment your have in your hands an evidence-based remedy for the obesity epidemic. If you meet a victim of the disease, lend them your copy of this book. Write to your local paper. Twitter. Get in touch with the friends you meet on social websites. Become an unpaid counsellor whenever your advice is sought. The best way to learn is to teach. This carries its own reward, for you are what you give, not what you're given. Spread the good news. Post a blog. Start a self-help slimming club. Don't be deterred by setbacks. If you have long-term goals you won't be deterred by short-term failures. Be passionate in your outlook, for it's only when words are delivered from the heart that they enter the ear and touch the soul. There's nothing like a reformed alcoholic to help other topers overcome their addiction to drink, and the same applies to people who've successfully shed their surplus weight and can provide living proof that obesity can be overcome. Share your experience, and become an active participant in the global campaign to put an end to the obesity pandemic.

Children in Need

Most important of all, please do your utmost to help the overweight children in your family and local community. They are our future, and the ones who most desperately need our help. In Canada, in a single decade at the end of the twentieth century, the rates of obesity in boys nearly tripled. Being too busy to spend quality time with their children, many parents demonstrate their love by giving them candy and lashings of pocket money so they can buy Coke and cookies throughout the day. However frenetic our lives may be we have a duty to teach them how to live, and the most valuable gift we can give our family and friends is a good example. I'm appalled today to notice how many opinion formers – especially nurses, teachers and doctors – are visibly overweight. If children grow up in an environment where their teachers are fat, their parents are fat, and a high percentage of the adults waddling past them on the pavements are grossly obese, can one be surprised that they too become obese? And how in all conscience can health professionals offer advice about the prevention and treatment of obesity-related disease if they themselves are overweight? I'm as suspicious of fat doctors as I am of unhappy psychotherapists, impoverished stockbrokers and crooked priests.

The Great Divide

We have a duty to our children, and also to the world's poor and undernourished people. It's an untenable humanitarian crime that while millions in the developed world are dying of gluttony and greed, millions more in the Third World countries are dying of starvation. I've pledged to give whatever royalties I receive from the UK sales of this book to charities devoted to helping the malnourished in Ethiopia and sub-Saharan Africa. My pious hope is that a sprinkling of the people who benefit from the EssVee programme will spare a thought for those less fortunate than themselves, and give them the benefit of their counsel and care, and maybe make a contribution to a charity dedicated to serving their needs, using some of the money they've saved by curtailing their expenditure on junk foods and take-away meals. The more we share, the more we'll gain and the more our communities will flourish. This may initially be a laborious process, but eventually a tipping point will be reached when, having reached the state of critical mass, the campaign will gain strength and undergo a surge of exponential growth until the obesity plague is finally put to rout. By your own example you can be a catalyst for change, and help to bring about the lifestyle renaissance which the world so desperately needs. Then we can close the great divide between the haves and have-nots, by replacing gluttony and greed with caring, sharing and mutual support.

Acknowledgements

I am indebted to the countless doctors, psychologists and scientists whose pioneering research work I have studied over the past forty years. It is impossible to mention them by name, but their tireless endeavours form the scientific basis of this book, which is merely a bouquet created from the myriad flowers that they have grown. I also wish to acknowledge my lifetime indebtedness to Diana Tyler, the founder of MBA Literary Agents, who has been my UK mentor and guardian for over forty years. The same personal tribute and thanks are due to Al Zuckerman, the founder of Writers House, one of the world's most prodigious literary agencies, who has looked after my American and Canadian interests since 1976. Unstinting tribute must also be paid to Miles Bailey, the founder of the Choir Press, who has been responsible for the design and production of the book; and to Ned Benjamin who has been the dependable, modest mastermind behind the design and hosting of my two websites. And finally, I wish to acknowledge the steadfast and unwavering support I've received from my beloved wife, in this and every other venture of our joint lives.

Resources

Sporting chance

Obesity is a relatively recent affliction. To a very large extent it's the aftermath of the Industrial Revolution, which substituted horse power for muscle power. Nowadays we can spend an entire day doing little more energetic that turning the ignition key of a car. As a result our bodies get flabby and fat. Somehow we must find space in our frenetic daily lives to get more exercise. Most people find this is best done, or at least with greatest enjoyment, by taking part in sport. This blows away cares and worries, firms up the figure and makes sure that our bodies have an optimum level of muscle tissue, which consumes three times as many calories as a similar weight of fat – even when we're fast asleep!

Choose a sport which really gives you pleasure, and which you can pursue on a regular basis with minimum fuss and wasted travelling time. Today there's an embarrassment of choice. Some sports are clearly more energetic than others. For example, to burn up 200 calories you'd need to potter gently in the garden for 45 minutes, whereas you'd expend the same amount of energy with just 30 minutes energetic dancing or 25 minutes of squash. In the same way brisk walking burns up two thirds more energy than gentle walking. But don't bother about the mathematics. Just go out and have fun. Get yourself fit for life.

Here are some options for you to consider, with contact details of the ruling bodies of each sport so you can find your nearest activity centre. Now it's up to you. Get fit for life.

Archery
Archery GB
www.archerygb.org
enquiries@archerygb.org
Tel 01952 606019

Badminton
Badminton England
www.badmintonengland.co.uk
enquiries@badmintonengland.co.uk
Tel: 01908 268400

Cricket
English Cricket Board
www.play-cricket.com
playcricket@ecb.co.uk

Cycling
Cyclists' Tourist Club
www.ctc.org.uk
cycling@ctc.org.uk
Tel: 0844 736 8450

Fencing
British Fencing
www.britishfencing.com
headoffice@britishfencing.com
Tel: 020 8742 3032

Football
Amateur Football Alliance
www.amateur.fa.com
info@amateur-fa.com
Tel:020 8733 2613

Health Clubs
Virgin Active Health Clubs
www.virginactive.co.uk
Tel: 0207 717 9000
David Lloyd Health clubs
www.davidlloyd.co.uk
Tel: 0845 2176464

Hockey
England Hockey
www.englandhockey.co.uk
info@englandhockey.co.uk
Tel: 01628 897500

Horse riding
British Horse Society
www.bhs.org.uk
Tel: 02476 840518

Karate
Karate England
www.karateengland.org.uk
admin@karateengland.org.uk
Tel: 07931 545924

Keep fit
Keep Fit
www.keepfit.org.uk
kfa@emdp.org
Tel: 01403 266000
Fitness League
www.thefitnessleague.com
info@thefitnessleague.com
Tel: 01344 874787

Netball
English Netball Association
www.englandnetball.co.uk
info@englandnetball.co.uk
Tel: 01462 442344

Orienteering
British Orienteering
www.britishorienteering.org.uk
info@britishorienteering.org.uk
Tel: 0161 2314499

Pilates
Pilates
www.pilates.co.uk

Rambling
Rambler's Association
www.ramblers.org.uk
ramblers@ramblers.org.uk
Tel: 020 7339 8500

Rugby
Rugby Football Union
www.rfu.com
community@therfu.com
British Amateur Rugby League
Association
www.barla.org.uk
info@barla.org.uk
Tel: 01484 544131

Squash
English Squash and Racket Ball
www.englandsquashandracketball.com
enquiries@englandsquashandracketball.com
Tel: 0161 2314499

Swimming
Amateur Swimming Association
www.swimming.org
customerservices@swimming.org
Tel: 01509 618700

Table Tennis
English Table Tennis Association
www.etta.tv
admin@etta.co.uk
Tel: 01424 722525

Tennis
Lawn Tennis Association
www.lta.org.uk
info@LTA.org.uk
Tel: 020 8487 7000

Volleyball
English Volleyball Association
www.volleyballengland.org
info@volleyballengland.org
Tel: 01509 227722

Spread the news! Become an agent of change. If you have drawn benefit from this book please tell your friends, by email, phone or word-of-mouth recommendation. Better still buy, and give them, a copy of the book. The Chinese have a saying 'When someone shares with you something of value, you have an obligation to share it with others.' This caring act could save their life, for anyone who sheds twenty pounds and retains that weight loss, cuts their overall mortality risk by a quarter.

To order a copy of the book online, and have it dispatched to any address in the UK, visit the website of the Self Health Alliance, and fill in the form which is prominently displayed on http://selfhelpalliance.co.uk/categegory/obesity. The Self Help Alliance is a not-for-profit organisation, which is running a campaign in 2012 to tackle the UK obesity plague. This is being run in conjunction with the London Olympics, and aims to encourage people of all ages, who are inspired by the spirit of the games and the performance of the world's elite athletes, to improve their personal fitness levels so that by the end of the year they too can take their place on the winner's rostrum. This, we believe, would be the finest possible legacy of the UK Olympiad. I've pledged to give whatever royalties I receive from the online sales of the book to charities providing nourishment, health care and clean water supplies to under-privileged communities in Somalia and sub-Saharan Africa.